New Insights into Contraception

New Insights into Contraception

Editors

**Giuseppe Benagiano
Francesco Maria Primiero**

MDPI • Basel • Beijing • Wuhan • Barcelona • Belgrade • Manchester • Tokyo • Cluj • Tianjin

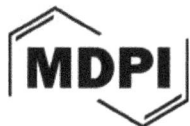

Editors
Giuseppe Benagiano
Sapienza University of Rome
Italy

Francesco Maria Primiero
Sapienza University of Rome
Italy

Editorial Office
MDPI
St. Alban-Anlage 66
4052 Basel, Switzerland

This is a reprint of articles from the Special Issue published online in the open access journal *Journal of Clinical Medicine* (ISSN 2077-0383) (available at: https://www.mdpi.com/journal/jcm/special_issues/Contraception).

For citation purposes, cite each article independently as indicated on the article page online and as indicated below:

LastName, A.A.; LastName, B.B.; LastName, C.C. Article Title. *Journal Name* **Year**, *Volume Number*, Page Range.

ISBN 978-3-0365-7276-5 (Hbk)
ISBN 978-3-0365-7277-2 (PDF)

© 2023 by the authors. Articles in this book are Open Access and distributed under the Creative Commons Attribution (CC BY) license, which allows users to download, copy and build upon published articles, as long as the author and publisher are properly credited, which ensures maximum dissemination and a wider impact of our publications.

The book as a whole is distributed by MDPI under the terms and conditions of the Creative Commons license CC BY-NC-ND.

Contents

Giuseppe Benagiano and Francesco M. Primiero
Special Issue "New Insights into Contraception"
Reprinted from: *J. Clin. Med.* **2022**, *11*, 6651, doi:10.3390/jcm11226651 1

Fatima Leon-Larios, José Gutiérrez Ales, María José Puente Martínez, Marta Correa Rancel, Isabel Lahoz Pascual, Isabel Silva Reus and José Cruz Quílez Conde
Results of the National Contraception Survey Conducted by *Sociedad Española de Contracepción* (2020)
Reprinted from: *J. Clin. Med.* **2022**, *11*, 3777, doi:10.3390/jcm11133777 5

Anna M. Jambrina, Pilar Rius, Pilar Gascón, Mercè Armelles, Mariona Camps-Bossacoma, Àngels Franch and Manel Rabanal
Characterization of the Use of Emergency Contraception from Sentinel Pharmacies in a Region of Southern Europe
Reprinted from: *J. Clin. Med.* **2021**, *10*, 2793, doi:10.3390/jcm10132793 19

Fatima Leon-Larios, Cecilia Ruiz-Ferron, Rocio-Marina Jalon-Neira and Juan-Manuel Praena-Fernández
Nursing Students' Knowledge, Awareness, and Experiences of Emergency Contraception Pills' Use
Reprinted from: *J. Clin. Med.* **2022**, *11*, 418, doi:10.3390/jcm11020418 31

Fatima Leon-Larios, Isabel Silva Reus, Isabel Lahoz Pascual, José Cruz Quílez Conde, María José Puente Martínez, José Gutiérrez Ales and Marta Correa Rancel
Women's Access to Sexual and Reproductive Health Services during Confinement Due to the COVID-19 Pandemic in Spain
Reprinted from: *J. Clin. Med.* **2022**, *11*, 4074, doi:10.3390/jcm11144074 41

Salvatore Caruso, Gaia Palermo, Giuseppe Caruso and Agnese Maria Chiara Rapisarda
How Does Contraceptive Use Affect Women's Sexuality? A Novel Look at Sexual Acceptability
Reprinted from: *J. Clin. Med.* **2022**, *11*, 810, doi:10.3390/jcm11030810 51

Aliye Runyan, Robert A. Welch, Katherine J. Kramer, Sarah Cortez, LeAnne J. Roberts, Clementina Asamoah, et al.
Long-Acting Reversible Contraception: Placement, Continuation, and Removal Rates at an Inner-City Academic Medical Center Clinic
Reprinted from: *J. Clin. Med.* **2021**, *10*, 1918, doi:10.3390/jcm10091918 63

Paola Bianchi, Sun-Wei Guo, Marwan Habiba and Giuseppe Benagiano
Utility of the Levonorgestrel-Releasing Intrauterine System in the Treatment of Abnormal Uterine Bleeding and Dysmenorrhea: A Narrative Review
Reprinted from: *J. Clin. Med.* **2022**, *11*, 5836, doi:10.3390/jcm11195836 73

Guglielmo Stabile, Carmelina Foti, Denise Mordeglia, Davide De Santo, Francesco Paolo Mangino, Antonio Simone Laganà and Giuseppe Ricci
Alternative Insertion Site of Nexplanon: Description of a Case Report and Systematic Review of the Literature
Reprinted from: *J. Clin. Med.* **2022**, *11*, 3226, doi:10.3390/jcm11113226 95

David F. Archer, Diana Mansour and Jean-Michel Foidart
Bleeding Patterns of Oral Contraceptives with a Cyclic Dosing Regimen: An Overview
Reprinted from: *J. Clin. Med.* **2022**, *11*, 4634, doi:10.3390/jcm11154634 103

Naama Vilk Ayalon, Lior Segev, Abraham O. Samson, Simcha Yagel, Sarah M. Cohen, Tamar Green and Hila Hochler
Norethisterone Reduces Vaginal Bleeding Caused by Progesterone-Only Birth Control Pills
Reprinted from: *J. Clin. Med.* **2022**, *11*, 3389, doi:10.3390/jcm11123389 . . . . **119**

Franca Fruzzetti, Tiziana Fidecicchi, Maria Magdalena Montt Guevara and Tommaso Simoncini
Estetrol: A New Choice for Contraception
Reprinted from: *J. Clin. Med.* **2021**, *10*, 5625, doi:10.3390/jcm10235625 . . . . **129**

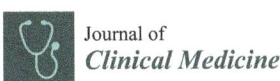

Journal of
Clinical Medicine

Editorial

Special Issue "New Insights into Contraception"

Giuseppe Benagiano [1,*] and Francesco M. Primiero [2]

1. Faculty of Medicine and Dentistry, Sapienza University of Rome, Policlinico Umberto I, Viale del Policlinico 115, 00161 Rome, Italy
2. Faculty of Medicine and Psychology, Sapienza University of Rome, Ospedale Sant'Andrea, Via di Grottarossa 1035/1039, 00189 Rome, Italy
* Correspondence: giuseppe.benagiano@fondazione.uniroma1.it

Citation: Benagiano, G.; Primiero, F.M. Special Issue "New Insights into Contraception". *J. Clin. Med.* **2022**, *11*, 6651. https://doi.org/10.3390/jcm11226651

Received: 4 November 2022
Accepted: 8 November 2022
Published: 9 November 2022

Publisher's Note: MDPI stays neutral with regard to jurisdictional claims in published maps and institutional affiliations.

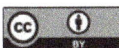

Copyright: © 2022 by the authors. Licensee MDPI, Basel, Switzerland. This article is an open access article distributed under the terms and conditions of the Creative Commons Attribution (CC BY) license (https://creativecommons.org/licenses/by/4.0/).

Today, a diverse range of contraceptive techniques is available to women; this, coupled with continued positive trends in female children and adults' educational attainment, will hasten declines in fertility and continue to slow population growth. With the advent of a sustained fertility rate lower than the replacement level in many countries, including China and India, we are already witnessing major economic, social, environmental, and geopolitical consequences [1].

Hormonal contraception, which was initially available as a daily pill, can be administered through seven different routes today: intramuscularly, intranasally, intra-uterus, intravaginally, orally, subcutaneously, and transdermally. New advancements have also been made in intrauterine contraception with the development of "frameless" devices. Last, but not least, research is being undertaken to provide effective emergency contraception after unprotected intercourse. The use of selective progesterone receptor modulators (antiprogestins) is very promising in this area [2].

The expansion of contraceptive use worldwide was a main priority during the second half of the twentieth century. As countries in the developed world (but also in a number of developing countries) reached and even went below the replacement level of fertility, issues regarding contraception seem to have been placed on the back burner.

Yet, since the milestone final declaration of the Cairo Conference on Population and Development in 1994 [3], contraception has been considered the main tool used for effective family planning, while at the same time, too much emphasis has been placed on 'technology' as the solution. Unfortunately, each advancement in technology has shown that every new or improved method carries side effects which are disturbing to some users. Clearly, there is no perfect method. In addition, at the field level, national and regional family-planning programs are far from being ideally run. This is why the utilization of new technology will depend on the way it is applied in the field. Focusing on the needs of women (and men) will remedy the errors of the past, when contraceptive development was exclusively driven by scientists, without the consideration of users' perspectives.

Because of this reality, the universal acceptance of methods of family planning, the best measure to prevent voluntary interruption of pregnancy (VIP), necessitates an integrated approach. Contraception must therefore be included in the broader concept of Sexual and Reproductive Health. This means that family planning and contraception must be placed within the wider paradigm of health, the health of the mother, and the health of her child. This in turn must be accepted as a task for individual couples, being a health and development issue, not a demographic one.

Promoting the use of contraception within the framework of improving health, not demography, means placing the emphasis on individuals, not methods alone, and on quality of services, not simply on availability through better distribution. Indeed, there is increasing awareness that contraception can help women to reduce health risks associated with reproductive events and specifically with unwanted pregnancies. In conclusion, no matter how ideal a method may be considered from a purely scientific viewpoint, it will be challenged by the constraints of the system in which it will be applied.

To contribute to the new *user-centered* perspective, the present issue of the *Journal of Clinical Medicine* presents a series of articles in which technology is considered within the broader concept of women's health.

To begin with, five articles deal with issues related to users' and providers' perspectives. The first reported on a National Contraception Survey conducted to explore the sexual and contraceptive habits of 1801 Spanish women of reproductive age [4]. Among those enrolled in the study, 78.7% used some kind of contraceptive method; the most frequently utilized were condoms (31.3%) and combined oral contraceptives (COCs) (18.5%). Interestingly, one fourth of the participants used both condoms and a COC; the majority of these participants were younger women and those with no steady partners. The investigation found that health professionals have an important role in the choice of a method, although less so with teenagers. Finally, the survey found that emergency contraception (EC) is increasingly being used, especially among those not using contraception on a regular basis.

With regard to EC, a second investigation [5] tried to gather information regarding the profiles of users in Catalonia, Spain, finding that 44.2% of respondents were 'repeat' users, and among them, 56.7% used a barrier method; more than 40% of couples who had unprotected intercourse stated that they utilized a natural family-planning (NFP) method. The study concluded that there was still a high proportion of repeat users with risky sexual behaviors, highlighting the need to provide better information, education, and preventive strategies.

A third survey also from Spain [6], analyzed knowledge, attitude, and awareness towards EC among 478 nursing students at the University of Seville and found that all of them knew of the existence of EC and had a positive attitude towards this method. One fourth of responders had used the method, mainly because of condom failure, or because they did not use any form of contraception. The survey found improper knowledge of the mechanism of action, efficacy and repeated use, and the type of pills available. The authors concluded that further education initiatives should focus on the mode of use, efficacy, and mechanism of action.

Access to reproductive health and family-planning services during lockdowns in the COVID-19 pandemic was the subject of the fourth descriptive, cross-sectional study conducted in the Canary Islands (Spain) on a random sample stratified by age on a total of 1800 women (response rate: 98.72%) [7]. Given the difficulty of providing counseling in person, a telematic approach was also offered. This method did create access problems in one third of the cases, but it was considered an overall success, as it resulted in a considerable decrease in the recurrent use of both EC and services for the VIP. The survey evidenced the existence of cases of gender-based violence among women cohabitating with their aggressors during lockdowns.

The fifth report deals with an important question from users' perspective of utilizing a contraceptive, namely the possibility that a given method (be it hormonal, barrier, or intrauterine) may modify a woman's sexuality [8]. To explore this issue, the study provided an overview of the effects of different methods of contraception on female sexuality. It also summarized recent investigations in which a variety of positive and negative consequences of contraceptive use were described regarding several aspects of sexual functions (desire, arousal, orgasm, pain, and enjoyment), stressing that sexual satisfaction depends on factors that extend beyond sexual functioning alone.

Three of the published articles dealt with a modality that is gaining increasing amounts of attention: the so-called Long-Acting Reversible Contraception (LARC).

The first article presented the results of a retrospective electronic chart review of 311 insertions of either the levonorgestrel-releasing intrauterine device (LNG-IUS), or the subcutaneous etonogestrel implant (SEI) in a center in the USA [9]. Delays in insertion were found in 38% of the subjects, mostly because of the absence of a qualified provider or device availability. Teenage users favored the SEI, whereas older women preferred the LNG-IUS. Retention time varied by device type, and most subjects eventually switched to other contraceptives. No patients experienced expulsion of the system.

Some LARC methods, specifically the LNG-IUS, have been used for a variety of non-contraceptive indications; this was the subject of a review of the utility of the system in women with heavy menstrual bleeding and/or dysmenorrhea [10]. Data from the literature show accumulating evidence that the insertion of such a device represents a useful option for long-term treatment. As a consequence of bearing the system, there is an improvement in the quality of life, a reduction in menstrual blood loss superior to that obtainable with other medical therapies, and a decrease in the extent of dysmenorrhea and pelvic pain. The likely mechanism of action of the system seems to be its ability to induce amenorrhea, which effectively eliminates both symptoms.

An uncommon but important limitation in the use of the SEI is represented by social and psychiatric disorders, in which the ready accessibility of the device by the subject becomes a negative feature. To obviate this situation, a device was successfully inserted into the scapular region in a young woman with a chronic psychiatric disorder [11].

The last three contributions to this Special Issue dealt with new advancements in oral hormonal contraception (OHC).

An important unwanted effect in this field is bleeding irregularities, which is cited as one of the major reasons for the discontinuation of these methods, and therefore, bleeding irregularities have been the focus of numerous investigations. The first of the three articles regarding OHC in this issue provided an overview of bleeding data related to the recently marketed cyclic COC and one progestin-only pill (POP) [12]. In this study, data from recent trials carried out to gain regulatory approval was evaluated, and it was concluded that each type of OHC has its own specific bleeding pattern; unfortunately, methodological differences hampered a comparison between products. The first consideration is that the balance between the effects of progestin and estrogen on the endometrium, the key factor in producing a regular bleeding pattern, seems lost when using a too-low dose of ethinylestradiol (EE) in order to reduce the risk of venous thromboembolism. The recent attempt to replace EE by 17β-estradiol (E2) or E2 valerate may lead to a suboptimal bleeding profile due to endometrial destabilization. In an attempt to, if not eliminate, then at least decrease the occurrence of bleeding problems, it has been recently proposed to utilize a derivative of estriol, namely estetrol (15α-hydroxyestriol) (E4), a natural estrogen exclusively produced in the fetal liver, in combination with drospirenone (DRSP). This combination yields a predictable, regular bleeding profile. It is worth noting that when DRSP is employed alone, the resulting bleeding pattern becomes somewhat unpredictable, stressing the usefulness of adding an estrogen.

The issue of irregular bleeding patterns in POPs was discussed in the second article on OHC [13]. Starting from the fact that no effective solution to this problem has been found, the authors examined therapeutic options being offered by health providers through a prospective questionnaire comparing the effectiveness of various treatments. Different regimens were tested: (1) POPs with norethisterone; (2) double-dose POPs; (3) single-dose POPs; (4) different POP formulae. They found that women for whom 5 mg of norethisterone acetate was added reported a significant decrease in bleeding frequency compared to the other groups. This was associated with an overall decrease in bleeding quantity and frequency.

The last article in the series summarized the present state of a COC in which DRSP is combined with E4 [14]. Clinical studies show efficacy, bleeding patterns and tolerability comparable to those of preparations with EE, thus determining high acceptability and user satisfaction. In addition, minimal effects have been found on lipids, liver parameters, Sex Hormone Binding Globulin (SHBG), and carbohydrate metabolism. A possible lower risk of venous thromboembolism and a better cardiovascular safety profile need to be investigated in further, large-scale studies.

In conclusion, the field of contraception continues to expand in search for more acceptable and safer modalities and routes of administration. At the same time, today, increased attention is paid to users' perspective and needs. This new focus means the available methods must be made suitable for different categories of subjects, ranging from teenagers to pre-menopausal women.

Today, contraception is much more than a technology; it has been the major instrument of a true social revolution that led to a—now often unwelcome—continued low fertility rate, while at the same time enhancing female reproductive health. Finding a correct balance between these aspects will be crucial in the years to come.

Author Contributions: G.B. and F.M.P. drafted the text. All authors have read and agreed to the published version of the manuscript.

Funding: This research received no external funding.

Conflicts of Interest: The authors declare no conflict of interest.

References

1. Benagiano, G.; Bastianelli, C.; Farris, M. Contraception Today. *Ann. N. Y. Acad. Sci.* **2006**, *1092*, 1–32. [CrossRef] [PubMed]
2. Vollset, S.E.; Goren, E.; Yuan, C.-W.; Cao, J.; Smith, A.E.; Hsiao, T.; Bisignano, C.; Azhar, G.S.; Castro, E.; Chalek, J.; et al. Fertility, mortality, migration, and population scenarios for 195 countries and territories from 2017 to 2100: A forecasting analysis for the Global Burden of Disease Study. *Lancet* **2020**, *396*, 1285–1306. [CrossRef]
3. United Nations. *Programme of Action of the International Conference on Population and Development*; Document CAI. 94–297; United Nations: New York, NY, USA, 1994.
4. Leon-Larios, F.; Gutiérrez Ales, J.; Puente Martínez, M.J.; Correa Rancel, M.; Lahoz Pascual, I.; Silva Reus, I.; Quílez Conde, J.C. Results of the National Contraception Survey Conducted by Sociedad Española de Contracepción (2020). *J. Clin. Med.* **2022**, *11*, 3777. [CrossRef] [PubMed]
5. Jambrina, A.; Rius, P.; Gascón, P.; Armelles, M.; Camps-Bossacoma, M.; Franch, À.; Rabanal, M. Characterization of the Use of Emergency Contraception from Sentinel Pharmacies in a Region of Southern Europe. *J. Clin. Med.* **2021**, *10*, 2793. [CrossRef] [PubMed]
6. Leon-Larios, F.; Ruiz-Ferron, C.; Jalon-Neira, R.-M.; Praena-Fernández, J.-M. Nursing Students' Knowledge, Awareness, and Experiences of Emergency Contraception Pills' Use. *J. Clin. Med.* **2022**, *11*, 418. [CrossRef] [PubMed]
7. Leon-Larios, F.; Reus, I.S.; Pascual, I.L.; Conde, J.C.Q.; Martínez, M.J.P.; Ales, J.G.; Rancel, M.C. Women's Access to Sexual and Reproductive Health Services during Confinement Due to the COVID-19 Pandemic in Spain. *J. Clin. Med.* **2022**, *11*, 4074. [CrossRef] [PubMed]
8. Caruso, S.; Palermo, G.; Caruso, G.; Rapisarda, A.M.C. How Does Contraceptive Use Affect Women's Sexuality? A Novel Look at Sexual Acceptability. *J. Clin. Med.* **2022**, *11*, 810. [CrossRef] [PubMed]
9. Runyan, A.; Welch, R.; Kramer, K.; Cortez, S.; Roberts, L.; Asamoah, C.; Ottum, S.; Sanders, J.; Shafi, A.; Recanati, M.-A. Long-Acting Reversible Contraception: Placement, Continuation, and Removal Rates at an Inner-City Academic Medical Center Clinic. *J. Clin. Med.* **2021**, *10*, 1918. [CrossRef] [PubMed]
10. Bianchi, P.; Guo, S.-W.; Habiba, M.; Benagiano, G. Utility of the Levonorgestrel-Releasing Intrauterine System in the Treatment of Abnormal Uterine Bleeding and Dysmenorrhea: A Narrative Review. *J. Clin. Med.* **2022**, *11*, 5836. [CrossRef] [PubMed]
11. Stabile, G.; Foti, C.; Mordeglia, D.; De Santo, D.; Mangino, F.P.; Laganà, A.S.; Ricci, G. Alternative Insertion Site of Nexplanon: Description of a Case Report and Systematic Review of the Literature. *J. Clin. Med.* **2022**, *11*, 3226. [CrossRef] [PubMed]
12. Archer, D.F.; Mansour, D.; Foidart, J.-M. Bleeding Patterns of Oral Contraceptives with a Cyclic Dosing Regimen: An Overview. *J. Clin. Med.* **2022**, *11*, 4634. [CrossRef] [PubMed]
13. Ayalon, N.V.; Segev, L.; Samson, A.O.; Yagel, S.; Cohen, S.M.; Green, T.; Hochler, H. Norethisterone Reduces Vaginal Bleeding Caused by Progesterone-Only Birth Control Pills. *J. Clin. Med.* **2022**, *11*, 3389. [CrossRef] [PubMed]
14. Fruzzetti, F.; Fidecicchi, T.; Guevara, M.M.M.; Simoncini, T. Estetrol: A New Choice for Contraception. *J. Clin. Med.* **2021**, *10*, 5625. [CrossRef] [PubMed]

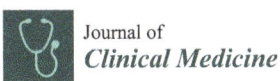

Article

Results of the National Contraception Survey Conducted by *Sociedad Española de Contracepción* (2020)

Fatima Leon-Larios [1], José Gutiérrez Ales [2], María José Puente Martínez [3,*], Marta Correa Rancel [4,5], Isabel Lahoz Pascual [6], Isabel Silva Reus [7] and José Cruz Quílez Conde [8]

[1] Nursing Department, University of Seville, 41004 Sevilla, Spain; fatimaleon@us.es
[2] Hospital Universitario Virgen Macarena, 41009 Sevilla, Spain; jgales050655@gmail.com
[3] Hospital San Pedro, 26006 Logroño, Spain
[4] Hospital Universitario de Canarias, 38320 Tenerife, Spain; tenerife1833@gmail.com
[5] Departamento de Obstetricia-Ginecología, Pediatría, Preventiva, Medicina Legal y Forense, Microbiología, Parasitología, Universidad de la Laguna, 38200 Santa Cruz de Tenerife, Spain
[6] Hospital Clínico Universitario Zaragoza, 50009 Zaragoza, Spain; isalahoz@yahoo.com
[7] Centro de Salud Sexual y Reproductiva de Villena, 03400 Alicante, Spain; isasilreus@gmail.com
[8] Hospital Universitario de Basurto, 48013 Bilbo, Spain; jotxe_c@hotmail.com
* Correspondence: mjpuente@riojasalud.es

Citation: Leon-Larios, F.; Gutiérrez Ales, J.; Puente Martínez, M.J.; Correa Rancel, M.; Lahoz Pascual, I.; Silva Reus, I.; Quílez Conde, J.C. Results of the National Contraception Survey Conducted by *Sociedad Española de Contracepción* (2020). *J. Clin. Med.* **2022**, *11*, 3777. https://doi.org/10.3390/jcm11133777

Academic Editors: Giuseppe Benagiano and Francesco Maria Primiero

Received: 18 May 2022
Accepted: 28 June 2022
Published: 29 June 2022

Publisher's Note: MDPI stays neutral with regard to jurisdictional claims in published maps and institutional affiliations.

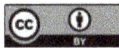

Copyright: © 2022 by the authors. Licensee MDPI, Basel, Switzerland. This article is an open access article distributed under the terms and conditions of the Creative Commons Attribution (CC BY) license (https://creativecommons.org/licenses/by/4.0/).

Abstract: Background: The National Contraception Survey conducted by *Sociedad Española de Contracepción* intends to know the sexual and contraceptive habits of Spanish women of reproductive age. Methods: A descriptive and cross-sectional study with random sample selection was conducted with women aged from 14 to 49 years old in July and August 2020. Results: A total of 1801 women participated in the study, of which 78.7% used some contraception method during their sexual relationships. The most frequently used methods were condoms (31.3%) and combined oral contraceptives (18.5%) at their last sexual encounter. A total of 25.7% used both condoms and pills, especially younger women and those who had no steady partners ($p < 0.001$). Use of Long-acting Reversible Contraceptives continues to be low, although a slight increase in their use is observed, and they are recommended for 50% of the users who need contraception. Counselling on contraception was provided to 64.3% of the women, mainly by their gynaecologists. Regarding the decision to use a contraceptive method, the one suggested by health professionals was more influential, although this was not the case for women aged less than 20 years old ($p < 0.001$). A total of 38.4% of the women have used emergency oral contraception at least once and 66.8% of those who do not make continuous use of contraception methods do so out of personal choice. Conclusions: It is necessary to deepen work on counselling and awareness among the population towards the use of efficient contraceptive methods that prevent unplanned pregnancies.

Keywords: contraception; sexual habits; women; long-acting reversible contraceptives; short-acting reversible contraceptives; counselling; emergency contraception

1. Introduction

Age at sexual debut has gradually dropped in the new generations [1,2], which is one reason why it has become necessary to implement adequate sexual and contraceptive counselling and provide information that prevents unintended pregnancies and sexually transmitted infections [3]. The rate of unwanted pregnancies in Spain continues to be higher than desired [4]. According to the European Contraception Atlas, almost 4 out of 10 women undergo unplanned pregnancies [5], a reality that is similar to that of other countries such as France with 33.3% [2,6], Sweden with 22% [7] and the United Kingdom with one out of five pregnancies [3], although slightly lower than in the United States, where half of the women stated not having planned their pregnancies [8]. It is therefore deduced that a large part of the population does not have their contraceptive needs met.

The unmet need for contraception presents high figures in Spain [5], exceeding those of other European countries such as France with less than 3% [9], Sweden with 8.9% [7] or Great Britain with 12.4% [3,10], although it is a more pressing problem in developing countries [11].

The use of the most frequent contraceptive methods has remained relatively unchanged throughout the years. Despite the recommendations, condoms and pills are still the most used methods worldwide [3,11–13]. It has been widely proved that Long-acting Reversible Contraceptives (LARCs) are effective in the prevention of unwanted pregnancies, abortion or recurrent abortions, although their rate of use is below desired [3,14,15]. Previous studies have already indicated the need to favour access to LARCs meeting women's individual characteristics [16], regardless of factors such as education and income levels, marital status, or ethnicity [17,18].

Health education actions in terms of sexuality and contraception are increasingly implemented, and this can either exert an influence on the users' behaviours or not [19–21]. A number of already published studies indicate that the decision to use a given contraceptive method over another is usually influenced by the advice of a health professional [22,23]. In addition, there are factors that can exert an influence on the choice and use of one method over another. Some of these factors are education level, income level and religious beliefs, among others [20,24,25]. Therefore, it is necessary to consider them when individualized counselling is provided to the user.

Counselling is offered during consultations by nurses, midwives, primary care physicians and gynaecologists, although only the latter two are authorized to write medical prescriptions [22]. Access to contraceptive methods in Spain is affordable, considering that some of them are fully funded by the National Health System. However, access to counselling on contraception and sexual education are not uniformly egalitarian throughout the country, as they depend on regional policies [19]. Thus, while they are practically fully funded in some regions, there are deficits in others [26].

The main objective of this study was to understand the habits of the Spanish female population in relation to the use of contraceptive methods and sexual health. We are interested in determining the factors that favour the use of some methods over others in order to design strategies that allow an increase in the use of contraceptive methods and thus avoid unplanned pregnancies.

2. Materials and Methods

2.1. Study Design

A descriptive and cross-sectional study. This study is an analysis of the National Contraception Survey conducted by *Sociedad Española de Contracepción* every 2 years through SigmaDos, an international Marketing and Public Survey Study company headquartered in Spain.

2.2. Measures

An ad hoc questionnaire designed by health professionals specialized in contraception who are members of *Sociedad Española de Contracepción* was used. It includes data on the use of contraceptive methods as well as about the participants' sexual habits.

2.3. Data Collection

The survey was conducted via telephone calls by means of a structured questionnaire consisting of 31 questions related to the interviewees' sexual and reproductive health. It was conducted from 31 July to 15 August 2020.

2.4. Sample Size

The women included were those of reproductive age between 14 and 49 years old throughout Spain. Sample distribution was proportional to that of the Spanish actual population, with an adjustment system by age quotas, in which the last interviewee selection instance was fully random. This distribution allowed offering representative data at the national level, although not at the level of geographical regions or areas.

Sample size was 1801 participants, with a possible error of +2.35% for a 95.5% confidence level.

2.5. Data Analysis

A univariate and bivariate analysis was performed to evaluate and know sexual behaviours and use of contraceptive methods in women of reproductive age. The χ^2 test was used to understand the relationship between use of the contraceptive methods and the sociodemographic characteristics, reporting φ as an indicator of size effect. The chi-square test was used to understand the relationship between use of the contraceptive methods and sociodemographic characteristics. A multivariate logistic regression was performed to find out the relationship between different variables. The results of the regression analysis were presented in terms of adjusted Odds Ratio (OR_{adj}), with a 95% confidence interval and significance level. Interpretation of the adjusted Odds Ratio can be as follows: if $OR_{adj} > 1$, then there are higher odds of using contraceptives.

In all hypothesis contrasts, the significance level was set at 0.05. Data analysis was processed in IBM SPSS 26 (IBM Corp., Armonk, NY, USA).

2.6. Ethical Aspects

This questionnaire was answered anonymously and ensuring the confidentiality of the participants. The women were free to stop answering questions at any moment. The Spanish health authorities do not require approval by a Research Ethics Committee for this type of study in which the participants are asked to provide data about their sexual and contraceptive practices outside a health environment that establishes a professional relationship. Verbal informed consent was requested from the participants at the beginning of the study.

3. Results

A total of 1801 women took part in the study, with a final response rate of 98.72%, which represents 1778 women. The participants' sociodemographic characteristics are presented in Table 1.

Table 1. Sociodemographic characteristics.

Variables	Total n (%) 1778 (100)
Age	
15–19 years old	170 (9.6)
20–24 years old	189 (10.6)
25–29 years old	211 (11.9)
30–34 years old	249 (14)
35–39 years old	308 (17.3)
40–44 years old	335 (18.8)
45–49 years old	316 (17.8)
Relationship situation	
Lives with her partner	1011 (56.9)
Steady partner, but not living together	325 (18.3)
No steady partner	442 (24.9)
Schooling level	
Elementary School	84 (4.7)
High School	917 (51.9)
University Studies	767 (43.4)

Table 1. Cont.

Variables	Total n (%) 1778 (100)
Nationality	
Spanish	1602 (90.2)
Other	174 (9.8)
Income level	
Low	401 (25.8)
Average-Low	663 (42.6)
Average	300 (19.3)
High	191 (12.3)
Work situation	1748 (100)
Working	1036 (59.3)
Not working	711 (40.7)
Religious beliefs	
Practicing Catholic	242 (13.6)
Lapsed Catholic	753 (42.4)
Other religions	111 (6.2)
Agnostic/Atheist	673 (37.8)

3.1. Sexual Habits

In total, 95.46% of the women aged between 15 and 49 years old had already engaged in sexual relationships at least once (16 years old is the minimum age for sexual consent). Globally, the mean age at the first sexual relationship was 18.07 years old. The age at the time of their first sexual relationship fluctuates between 19.83 years old in the case of the women aged between 45 and 49 years old and 15.83 years old in those aged between 15 and 19, as can be seen in Figure 1.

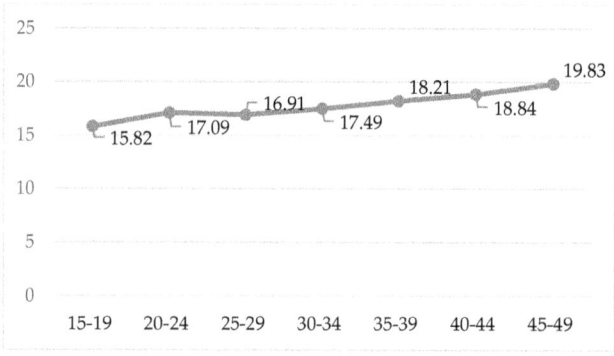

Figure 1. Age at the first sexual relationship according to age group.

Of the total of participating women, 89.8% engaged in sexual relationships with one of the frequencies shown in Figure 2, with determination that the higher the age, the lower the monthly frequency of sexual relationships: $\chi^2(18) = 61.56$, $p < 0.001$, $\varphi = 0.190$.

Out of all the women, 91.9% stated that they had engaged in sexual relationships in the last 12 months; on the other hand, 3.7% had already had sexual relationships at some moment in their life, although not in the last year. The mean number of sex partners during the last year was 1.36, being slightly higher among women aged less than 30 years old, as follows: from 15 to 19 years old, 1.71 partners; from 20 to 24 years old, 1.53; and from 25 to 29 years old, 1.51.

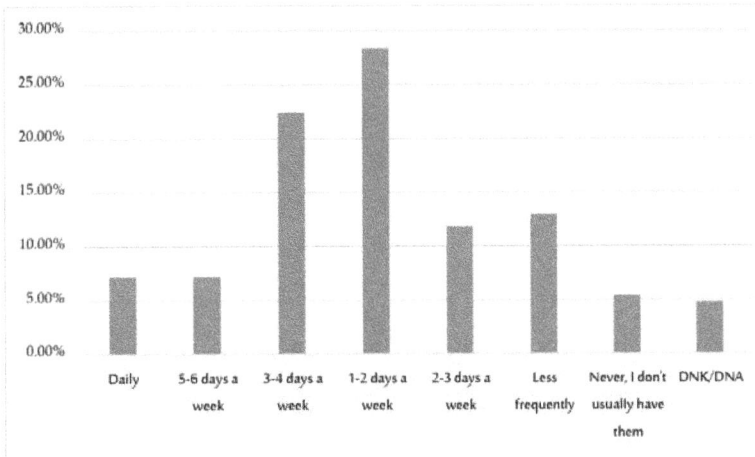

Figure 2. Frequency of sexual relationships.

Sexual Relationships and Use of Contraceptive Methods

When the women were asked if they have engaged in sexual relationships without contraceptive protection, 61.4% answered never and 15.8%, almost never. 21.3% reported having had sexual relationships with no contraceptive protection quite frequently, with a higher percentage in the age group from 30 to 34 years old, reaching 26.8%. Likewise, those women that lived with their partners (26.8%) and were Spanish (21.7%) were more likely to engage in sexual relationships without using any contraceptive method: $\chi^2(4) = 12.64$, $p = 0.013$, $\varphi = 0.091$.

The women at risk of unwanted pregnancies represented 22.9% of those that did not use any contraceptive method, accounting for 6.2% of the total women of reproductive age.

3.2. Use of Emergency Oral Contraception

In total, 38.4% of the women of reproductive age interviewed stated having consulted at some point about emergency oral contraception products that are dispensed free of charge in pharmacies at some moment. This percentage is higher in the age group from 20 to 39 years old, as shown in Figure 3.

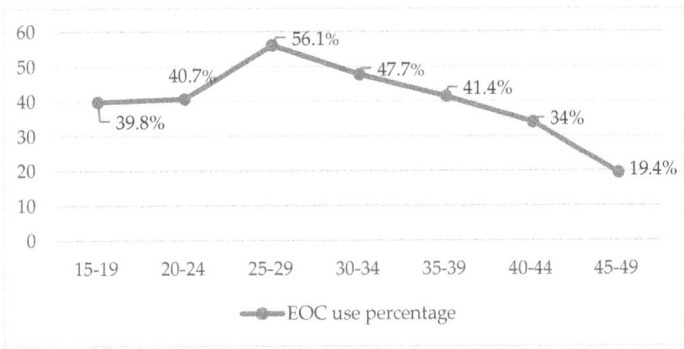

Figure 3. Use of the morning-after pill according to age group.

Use of the morning-after pill is more frequent in women that do not live with their partners (46.1%) [$\chi^2(4) = 23.51$, $p < 0.001$, $\varphi = 0.118$] or do not have a steady partner (43.4%) [$\chi^2(4) = 78.88$, $p = 0.008$, $\varphi = 0.216$], as well as among those who resort to condoms as their usual contraceptive method (46.8%) [$\chi^2(15) = 25.59$, $p = 0.043$, $\varphi = 0.153$], as shown in Table 2.

Table 2. Use of Emergency Contraception Pills (ECPs) over lifetime according to usual contraceptive method, nationality and relationship status.

Use of ECPs	Total	Relationship Situation			Contraceptive Methods Generally Used							Nationality	
		Lives with Her Partner	Steady Partner, Not Living Together	No Steady Partner	Condoms	Pills	IUD	Voluntary Sterilization	Other Methods	None		Spanish	Other
Yes	38.4%	34.1%	46.1%	43.4%	46.8%	40.8%	37.7%	30.0%	46.4%	30.2%		38.3%	39.8%
No	61.5%	65.9%	5.9%	56.3%	53.2%	59.2%	62.3%	70.0%	53.6%	69.8%		61.7%	60.2%
DNK/DNA	0.1%	0.0%	0.0%	0.3%	0.0%	0.0%	0.0%	0.0%	0.0%	0.0%		0.0%	0.0%

3.3. Information and Counselling on Contraceptive Methods

Most of the women (64.3%) consulted their primary care physician, gynaecologist, midwife or Family Planning Centre to receive counselling and therefore choose the method that best fitted their personal circumstances. The women belonging to the oldest age group attended health centres more frequently to receive individualized counselling: $\chi^2(12) = 83.39$, $p < 0.001$, $\varphi = 0.217$). It was noticed that the youngest women attended the centres in a lower proportion (37.8% of those aged less than 20 years old).

The contraceptive methods used by the women were as follows: the one indicated by the gynaecologist (42.4%), self-prescription (39.5%), the one suggested by the family physician (12.1%), a midwife/nurse (1.7%) and a pharmacist (0.6%). When the women were asked who was most influential on the definite choice of the method used, 44.2% stated that it was the health personnel, 31.2% indicated that it was their own decision, in 17.2% it was family members/friends, 2.4% mentioned the communication media, 1.9% pointed to social networks/Internet, 1.9% chose Others and 1.3% selected Does Not Know/Does Not Answer.

The health staff exerts less influence on the final decision about using one method over another, especially in those aged less than 20 years old, among which family members and friends are the most influential people (40.4%). If we perform an analysis according to the method used, it is observed that the women who chose oral combined hormonal contraception (69.3%) or IUD (60.9%) were driven by the influence exerted by a health professional. Personal choice for their use (42.3%) predominated among those who used condoms.

Not attending the consultation to receive counselling was not related to the schooling and income levels or to the religious beliefs but to nationality: $\chi^2(2) = 8.22$, $p = 0.016$, $\varphi = 0.068$, as can be seen in Table 3.

Table 3. Counselling on contraception over lifetime according to nationality, schooling and income levels and religious beliefs.

Counselling	Total	Nationality		Schooling Level			Income Level			Religious Beliefs			
		Spanish	Other	Elementary School	High School	University Studies	Low	Average-Low	Average	High	Practicing Catholic	Lapsed Catholic	Professes Other Religions	Agnostic/Atheist
Yes	64.3%	65.5%	54.6%	57.7%	64.2%	65.8%	63.3%	66.7%	71.4%	62.7%	62.6%	65.7%	59.3%	64.3%
No	35.6%	34.5%	45.4%	42.3%	35.8%	34.2%	36.7%	33.3%	28.6%	37.3%	37.4%	34.2%	40.7%	35.7%
DNK/DNA	0.0%	0.0%	0.0%	0.0%	0.1%	0.0%	0.0%	0.1%	0.0%	0.0%	0.0%	0.1%	0.0%	0.0%

Information and Counselling about Long-Acting Reversible Methods

In total, 49.9% of the women aged between 15 to 49 years old stated having been advised and offered information about some long-acting method (IUD or implant) at some moment. It was observed that it is more frequently offered to the oldest age group: $\chi^2(12) = 44.65, p < 0.001, \varphi = 0.158$, as can be seen in Figure 4.

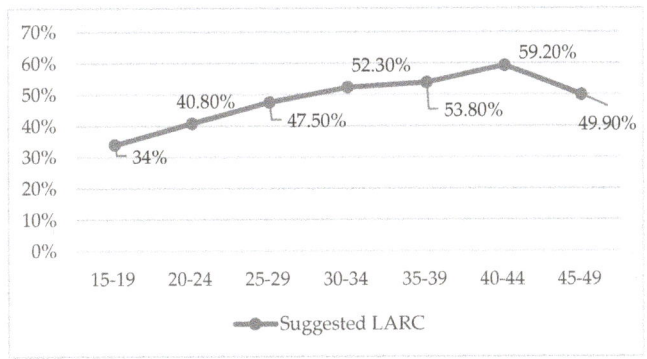

Figure 4. Counselling for the use of LARCs according to age group.

When the women were asked about the advantages perceived in using long-acting contraception methods, convenience was signalled as the main advantage of their use. 47.3% of the women aged between 15 and 49 years old identified this quality. Contraceptive efficacy (26.8%) was identified in the second place, while the greater safety offered by these contraceptive methods was ranked third (25.1%).

3.4. Contraceptive Use Pattern

It was found that 7 out of 10 Spanish women of reproductive age used some contraceptive method. It is to be considered that, among the women who did not resort to any contraceptive method are those that did not engage in sexual relationships while the study was conducted.

The age group that made the most use of some method during sexual relationships is the one from 20 to 30 years old, as can be seen in Figure 5.

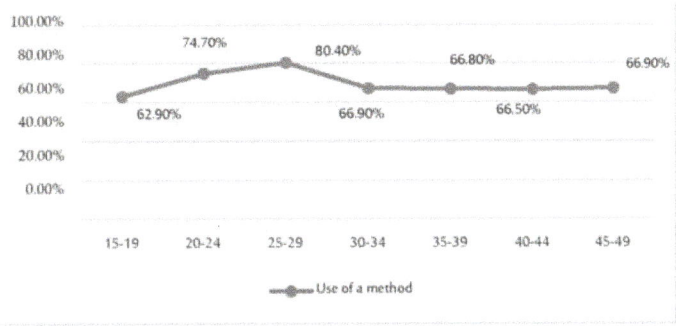

Figure 5. Use of some contraceptive method according to age group.

In relation to other analysis variables, it is worth noting the increase in the number of women who did not use any contraceptive method among those with lower income levels (33.9%) and those who are Catholics (32.2%); with this rate increasing especially with women who already have children and want more (41.8%): $\chi^2(6) = 28.50, p < 0.001, \varphi = 0.130$.

Condoms are the contraceptive method most frequently used (31.3%) by the women of reproductive age who engage in sexual relationships and use some method. Combined oral hormonal contraception ranks second (18.5%), followed by copper IUD (4.3%) and hormonal IUD (4.2%). Table 4 presents the contraceptive methods used by age groups from the total of women between 15 and 49 years old participating in the study. Condoms continue to be the most frequently used method in all age groups, and pills reach their maximum use value between the ages of 20 and 24, subsequently decreasing as age advances.

Table 4. Distribution of the use of contraceptive methods.

Effective methods (98.5%)	Barrier	Condoms		47.5%
	Hormonal (36%)	Oral administration (29.1%)	Pills	28.1%
			Mini pills	1.0%
		Intravaginal administration	Vaginal ring	3.2%
			Patch	1.0%
		Injectable (monthly-quarterly)		0.5%
		Subcutaneous implant (1 or 2 bars)		2.2%
	IUD (12.5%)	Copper		6.5%
		Hormone release		6.0%
	Voluntary sterilization (irreversible) 2.5%	Fallopian tube ligation/Essure procedure (tubal obstruction)		1.6%
		Vasectomy		0.9%
Little effective methods (0.2%)	Natural or Periodic abstinence	Knauss–Ogino (standard day method), Billings' method (cervical mucus), temperature method		0.1%
	Interruption	Coitus interruptus (withdrawal)		0.1%
Others				0.7%

Considering the different contraceptive methods and their characteristics, it is worth noting that 69.6% of the women of reproductive age used effective methods, reaching 99% of those that consulted about some method. 31.3% used barrier methods, 23.8% consulted regarding hormonal methods and 8.3% employed some type of IUD, as shown in Table 4.

3.4.1. Drivers for the Use of Reversible Methods

Overall, the reasons stated by the women for using the short-acting reversible contraceptive methods (SARCs) were as follows: convenience (48.4%) for all age groups, safety (37.5%), lower impact on health (37.5%), lifestyle (16.1%), medical recommendation (14.4%), contraceptive efficacy (13.1%), economic reasons (3.1%), DNK/DNA (1.9%) and Others (1%).

3.4.2. Hormonal Methods

The hormonal methods were employed following medical recommendations (23.9%) and for regulation of the menstrual cycle (19.8%). Those women who showed reluctance to use hormonal methods argued risk of hormonal use (29.1%), side effects and/or health problems (28.7%).

3.4.3. Discontinuation of Hormonal Contraception

In total, 68.9% of the participating women that sought consultations about combined hormonal methods did not discontinue their use periodically. On the other hand, less than one-third did so, due to personal choice (66.8%) based on diverse information or recommendations. In total, 29.7% implemented periodic discontinuation due to the health recommendations provided by physicians, midwives or nurses. Discontinuation tends to be higher with advancing age, exceeding 30% from the age of 25. The women who used pills interrupted their contraception more often over lifetime [$\chi^2(12) = 139.11, p < 0.001, \varphi = 0.358$], as well as those that already had children [$\chi^2(4) = 50.98, p < 0.001, \varphi = 0.381$], as can be seen in Table 5.

Table 5. Discontinuation in the use of contraceptives according to nationality, schooling level and desire to conceive fulfilled.

Disconti-nuation	Total	Nationality		Schooling Level			Motherhood Situation			
		Spanish	Other	Elementary School	High School	University Studies	Has Children and Wants More	Has Children and Does Not Want More	Does Not Have Children but Wants to	Does Not Have Children and Does Not Want to
Yes	28.0%	28.7%	15.7%	19.2%	29.5%	26.5%	31.8%	31.5%	26.6%	26.2%
No	68.9%	68.2%	80.1%	75.9%	68.4%	69.0%	68.2%	65.7%	69.7%	70.3%
DNK/DNA	3.2%	3.1%	4.2%	4.9%	2.2%	4.5%	0.0%	2.8%	3.7%	3.5%

3.4.4. Use of the Dual Method

Of all the women of reproductive age that use contraceptive methods, 25.7% stated resorting to the dual method (condoms and hormonal method and/or IUD). The most usual dual method combination corresponded to that of condoms and pills (28.1%). This practice was more frequent among the youngest women (from 15 to 19 years old). 8.8% consulted about it occasionally (almost never/sometimes) and 16.9% did so always/almost always.

Habitual use of the dual method (*always/almost always*) was more frequent among the women who had no steady partners (26.7%): $\chi^2(10) = 60.51, p < 0.001, \varphi = 0.235$, as indicated in Table 6.

Table 6. Use of the dual method according to nationality, having a partner or not and schooling level.

	Total	Nationality		Schooling Level			Relationship Situation		
		Spanish	Other	Elementary School	High School	University Studies	Lives with Her Partner	Steady Partner, but Not Living together	No Steady Partner
Yes (Always/Almost always)	16.9%	17.1%	14.6%	22.6%	18.8%	14.6%	11.8%	20.5%	26.7%
No (Never, Almost never or Sometimes)	82.6%	82.4%	85.4%	75.1%	81.0%	84.8%	87.7%	79.5%	72.6%
DNK/DNA	0.4%	0.5%	0.0%	2.3%	0.1%	0.6%	0.5%	0.0%	0.7%

4. Discussion

This study intended to know the sexual behaviours and use patterns of contraceptive methods of women of reproductive age living in Spain. To such an end, this descriptive and cross-sectional study was conducted with a random and stratified sample of Spanish women of reproductive age in 2020.

Spanish women's age at the time of their first sexual relationship is estimated to be less than 18 years old. However, it is noticed that such age has been dropping according to the age groups. Women aged less than 20 years old initiated their sex lives four years earlier than their mothers, a finding that is in line with other European studies that estimate the age at the time of first sexual relationship to be 16 years old [2,7]. We have to be aware of the fact that women initiate their sex lives increasingly earlier in time; therefore, they have to resort to proper contraception methods if they want to avoid sexually transmitted infections or unwanted pregnancies; awareness of these methods can be achieved through sexual education [19,21].

The results obtained in this National Survey indicate that 7 out of 10 women use some type of contraceptive method. This is similar to the data contributed by other European studies [3,7], in which it was also already indicated that the higher the user's age, the lesser the use of contraceptive methods [27]. If we consider that the women that are at risk of unwanted pregnancies are those who, with the possibility of having children, do not want them and engage in sexual relationships without resorting to any contraceptive method, we would be talking about 2 out of 10 women. This tells us that, for this reason, it is still necessary to deepen work on prevention, especially in the extreme age groups: below 20 years old [28] and above 45 years old, which are the age groups where the highest use inconsistency is observed. More influence should be exerted on collective groups that respond to these premises, as counselling interventions turn out to be effective to increase contraceptive use and compliance rates [19,29].

Among the contraceptive methods most frequently used in women of reproductive age, condoms still rank first, followed by pills, although not only in Spain [12], as we notice the same trend if we investigate data published in other European countries [7,13]. Despite the increase in the use of hormonal methods, condoms are still the most frequent choice. However, their use decreases when women start to consider their partners as stable, a fact that has already been identified in similar studies [30]. The dual method is used, but especially in younger women, as the use of condoms is reduced as age advances [21]. Inconsistent condom use is related to late placement after intercourse has started; better condom use is noticeable in the youngest women (aged less than 19 years old), a fact that has not always been found in similar studies [31].

Counselling in terms of contraception is usually in charge of health professionals (family physicians, gynaecologists, midwives, nurses), although it is still more common for older women to attend contraceptive counselling appointments [32], reason why reinforcement is required in the youngest women regarding the need to receive information and guidance by duly qualified professionals, as already pointed out in previous studies [19,22]. The woman's choice regarding one method or another is influenced by the prescribing health professional, followed by her own personal criterion [22,33,34].

There is still a considerable number of women who resort to emergency oral contraception at some moment during their reproductive life, especially among those aged less than 40 years old [35]. Almost 4 out of 10 women have made use of emergency oral contraception at least once, a result that is in consonance with others published with young people belonging to similar age groups [4,36,37]. As was already pointed out by some studies, using it after a failure in the usual contraceptive method might contribute to reducing the number of unplanned pregnancies [4].

Despite its recommendation and of being a more economical option [26], the use of LARCs continues to be relatively low when compared to SARCs, a fact that has also been stated in studies conducted in other European countries such as Sweden, where 2 out of 10 women used LARCs [7]. It continues to be a more frequent contraception option in women aged over 30 years old [3].

Nevertheless, it was observed that counselling and the information provided about LARCs had increased, leading to an increase in their use when compared to previous years [3,13,38]. In addition, the recommendation to use them among the youngest women is increasingly frequent [39], as pointed out in our study. It is important that the family physicians and gynaecologists that will prescribe them know them, and be aware of and minimize personal bias for their recommendation [40]. In addition, when health professionals have sound knowledge of the method, they will better convey the information to the users, who will be able to choose it on better grounds. It has been shown that, when there are knowledge gaps, its use is lower among women [15,22], whereas when they know it in detail and know of someone who uses it, they consider it highly acceptable [41].

Among the main drivers for its use are safety and convenience, as well as prevention of unwanted pregnancies, as already pointed out by women participating in other similar studies [7]. Access and policies are usually important for the use of LARC methods. Those countries that have implemented policies that ensure availability and insertion of the device free of charge increase their use among women [16,42]. In our study, it has been noticed that many users underwent annual IUD control reviews, despite not being a specific recommendation [43], being more frequent in women with lower schooling levels.

On the other hand, a clear reduction is noticed in the habit of periodically discontinuing the use of hormonal methods. In 2014, 51% of the users who consulted about pills implemented intervals, with a progressive reduction until 2020, currently reaching 28%. Likewise, a difference is noticed in relation to previous years; it now responds to the women's own decisions rather than to a recommendation by a health professional [44]. This is in line with other studies conducted where a reduction in discontinuation of hormonal contraception was observed, although it is still used despite not being recommended, reason why work should be deepened to properly advise women [45].

5. Strengths and Limitations

One of the strengths of this study is the sample size achieved, which provides additional information with women from all regions and age groups, therefore allowing us to observe a real trend at the national level. As this is a cross-sectional study, we cannot establish causality, only associations between the variables defined. However, this study allows us to have a solid baseline of the reality regarding women's use of contraception and sexual behaviours in Spain.

This study was conducted during the pandemic that we are currently experiencing, therefore, its results must be interpreted considering this scenario. The results contributed by this National Contraception Survey were obtained during 2020; consequently, they are influenced by the situation experienced during the last two years in Europe after the declaration of the global pandemic, which may have affected the results.

6. Conclusions

The results found in this research allow focusing the attention on those women who are susceptible to not using consistent contraceptive methods. It allows defining the strategies for counselling by health professionals for the proper use of contraceptive methods that allow preventing unwanted pregnancies and abortions. It is necessary to continue developing strategies that reduce the unmet need for contraception in order to avoid unwanted pregnancies and continue working to identify the gaps that will allow for efficient counselling and adherence in the users, meeting their individual needs. It becomes necessary to keep fostering the use of LARCs in all age groups, not only in those women with their desire to conceive fulfilled or in those who belong to older age groups.

Author Contributions: Conceptualization and Methodology M.C.R., J.C.Q.C., I.S.R. and J.G.A. and Formal Analysis, F.L.-L. and I.L.P. Writing—Original Draft Preparation, F.L.-L., I.L.P., M.J.P.M., J.C.Q.C., M.C.R., J.C.Q.C., I.S.R. and J.G.A. All authors have read and agreed to the published version of the manuscript.

Funding: This research was funded by *Sociedad Española de Contracepción* (SEC). The APC was also funded by SEC.

Institutional Review Board Statement: This study did not require ethical approval. The study was conducted in accordance with the Declaration of Helsinki. Ethical review and approval were waived for this study due to participants being invited to participate voluntarily.

Informed Consent Statement: Informed consent was obtained from all subjects involved in the study prior to participation.

Data Availability Statement: The datasets that support the findings of this study are available from the corresponding author upon reasonable written request.

Acknowledgments: We would like to thank to the former board of *Sociedad Española de Contracepción* (SEC) their contribution to this research, especially Paloma Lobo Abascal, Jose Ramón Serrano Navarro and José Vicente González Navarro who participated in the design of the questionnaire. We also wish to thank *Sociedad Española de Contracepción* for their support to publish this paper.

Conflicts of Interest: The authors declare no conflict of interest. The funders had no role in the design of the study; in data collection, analyses or interpretation; in the writing of the manuscript; or in the decision to publish the results.

References

1. Young, H.; Burke, L.; Nic Gabhainn, S. Sexual intercourse, age of initiation and contraception among adolescents in Ireland: Findings from the Health Behaviour in School-aged Children (HBSC) Ireland study. *BMC Public Health* **2018**, *18*, 362. [CrossRef] [PubMed]
2. Jost, S.; Le Tohic, A.; Chis, C.; This, P.; Grosdemouge, I.; Panel, P. Contraception des femmes françaises de 15 à 45ans: Enquête nationale sur un échantillon représentatif de 5963 femmes [Contraception's choice: Women's opinion, satisfaction and profile. Results of a French national survey of a representative sample of 5963 women]. *Gynecol. Obstet. Fertil.* **2014**, *42*, 415–421. [CrossRef] [PubMed]
3. French, R.S.; Gibson, L.; Geary, R.; Glasier, A.; Wellings, K. Changes in the prevalence and profile of users of contraception in Britain 2000–2010: Evidence from two National Surveys of Sexual Attitudes and Lifestyles. *BMJ Sex. Reprod. Health* **2020**, *46*, 200–209. [CrossRef] [PubMed]
4. Lete, I.; Doval, J.L.; Pérez-Campos, E.; Alonso, M.J.; Sellers, G.; Sánchez-Borrego, R. Prevention of unintended pregnancies by using emergency contraception: The differences between levonorgestrel and ulipristal acetate. A theoretical model using data from a survey on the use of emergency contraception in Spain, 2017. *Gynecol. Endocrinol.* **2019**, *35*, 582–585. [CrossRef]
5. European Parliamentary Forum on Population & Development (EPF). CONTRACEPTION ATLAS. 2020. Available online: https://www.epfweb.org/european-contraception-atlas (accessed on 14 April 2022).
6. Bonnet, C.; Blondel, B.; Moreau, C. A rise in births following contraceptive failure in France between 2010 and 2016: Results from the French national perinatal surveys. *BMC Womens Health* **2021**, *21*, 115. [CrossRef]
7. Kopp Kallner, H.; Thunell, L.; Brynhildsen, J.; Lindeberg, M.; Gemzell Danielsson, K. Use of Contraception and Attitudes towards Contraceptive Use in Swedish Women—A Nationwide Survey. *PLoS ONE* **2015**, *10*, e0125990. [CrossRef]
8. Finer, L.B.; Zolna, M.R. Shifts in intended and unintended pregnancies in the United States, 2001–2008. *Am. J. Public Health* **2014**, *104* (Suppl. 1), S43–S48. [CrossRef]
9. Moreau, C.; Bohet, A.; Trussell, J.; Bajos, N. Estimates of unintended pregnancy rates over the last decade in France as a function of contraceptive behaviors. *Contraception* **2014**, *89*, 314–321. [CrossRef]
10. Alkema, L.; Kantorova, V.; Menozzi, C.; Biddlecom, A. National, regional, and global rates and trends in contraceptive prevalence and unmet need for family planning between 1990 and 2015: A systematic and comprehensive analysis. *Lancet* **2013**, *381*, 1642–1652. [CrossRef]
11. Blumenberg, C.; Hellwig, F.; Ewerling, F.; Barros, A.J.D. Socio-demographic and economic inequalities in modern contraception in 11 low- and middle-income countries: An analysis of the PMA2020 surveys. *Reprod. Health* **2020**, *17*, 82. [CrossRef]
12. Lete, I.; Dueñas-Díez, J.-L.; Martínez-Salmeán, J.; Parrilla, J.; Serrano, I.; Bermejo, R.; Coll, C.; Doval, J. Contraceptive practices and trends in Spain: 1997–2003. *Eur. J. Obstet. Gynecol. Reprod. Biol.* **2007**, *135*, 73–75. [CrossRef] [PubMed]
13. Podolskyi, V.; Gemzell-Danielsson, K.; Marions, L. Contraceptive experience and perception, a survey among Ukrainian women. *BMC Womens Health* **2018**, *18*, 159. [CrossRef] [PubMed]
14. Ihongbe, T.O.; Masho, S.W. Changes in the Use of Long-Acting Reversible Contraceptive Methods Among U.S. Nulliparous Women: Results from the 2006–2010, 2011–2013, and 2013–2015 National Survey of Family Growth. *J. Womens Health* **2018**, *27*, 245–252. [CrossRef] [PubMed]
15. Davis, S.A.; Braykov, N.P.; Lathrop, E.; Haddad, L.B. Familiarity with Long-acting Reversible Contraceptives among Obstetrics and Gynecology, Family Medicine, and Pediatrics Residents: Results of a 2015 National Survey and Implications for Contraceptive Provision for Adolescents. *J. Pediatr. Adolesc. Gynecol.* **2018**, *31*, 40–44. [CrossRef]
16. Ali, M.; Folz, R.; Farron, M. Expanding choice and access in contraception: An assessment of intrauterine contraception policies in low and middle-income countries. *BMC Public Health* **2019**, *19*, 1707. [CrossRef]
17. Beshar, I.; So, J.; Chelvakumar, M.; Cahill, E.P.; Shaw, K.A.; Shaw, J.G. Socioeconomic differences persist in use of permanent vs long-acting reversible contraception: An analysis of the National Survey of Family Growth, 2006 to 2010 vs 2015 to 2017. *Contraception* **2021**, *103*, 246–254. [CrossRef]
18. Grady, C.D.; Dehlendorf, C.; Cohen, E.D.; Schwarz, E.B.; Borrero, S. Racial and ethnic differences in contraceptive use among women who desire no future children, 2006–2010 National Survey of Family Growth. *Contraception* **2015**, *92*, 62–70. [CrossRef]
19. Diez, E.; Lopez, M.J.; Perez, G.; Garcia-Subirats, I.; Nebot, L.; Carreras, R.; Villalbi, J.R. Impact of a community contraceptive counselling intervention on adolescent fertility rates: A quasi-experimental study. *BMC Public Health* **2020**, *20*, 26. [CrossRef]

20. Liddon, N.; O'Malley Olsen, E.; Carter, M.; Hatfield-Timajchy, K. Withdrawal as pregnancy prevention and associated risk factors among US high school students: Findings from the 2011 National Youth Risk Behavior Survey. *Contraception* **2016**, *93*, 126–132. [CrossRef]
21. Jaramillo, N.; Buhi, E.R.; Elder, J.P.; Corliss, H.L. Associations Between Sex Education and Contraceptive Use Among Heterosexually Active, Adolescent Males in the United States. *J. Adolesc. Health* **2017**, *60*, 534–540. [CrossRef]
22. Harper, C.C.; Stratton, L.; Raine, T.R.; Thompson, K.; Henderson, J.T.; Blum, M.; Postlethwaite, D.; Speidel, J.J. Counseling and provision of long-acting reversible contraception in the US: National survey of nurse practitioners. *Prev. Med.* **2013**, *57*, 883–888. [CrossRef] [PubMed]
23. Lee, J.; Berenson, A.B.; Patel, P.R. Characteristics of Females Who Use Contraception at Coitarche: An Analysis of the National Survey of Family Growth 2006–2010 Database. *J. Womens Health* **2015**, *24*, 972–977. [CrossRef] [PubMed]
24. Daniels, K.; Abma, J.C. Current Contraceptive Status Among Women Aged 15–49: United States, 2017–2019. *NCHS Data Brief* **2020**, *388*, 1–8.
25. Lete, I.; Hassan, F.; Chatzitheofilou, I.; Wood, E.; Mendivil, J.; Lambreeli, D.; Filonenko, A.; Lambrelli, D. Direct costs of unintended pregnancy in Spain. *Eur. J. Contracept. Reprod. Health Care* **2015**, *20*, 308–318. [CrossRef] [PubMed]
26. Parra Ribes, I.; Rascón Poza, J.J.; Pérez Campos, E.; Bugella Yudice, I.; Rodríguez Domingo, M.J. Economic Burden of Contraception Management in Spain. *J. Health Econ. Outcomes Res.* **2018**, *6*, 63–74. [CrossRef]
27. Chuy, V.S.; Rajagopal, G.; Talluri, R.; Cheng, A.L. Factors Influencing Contraceptive Use Among Sexually Active U.S. Middle and High School Students, 2015 to 2019. *Cureus* **2021**, *13*, e20803. [CrossRef]
28. Scott, R.H.; Wellings, K.; Lindberg, L. Adolescent Sexual Activity, Contraceptive Use, and Pregnancy in Britain and the U.S.: A Multidecade Comparison. *J. Adolesc. Health* **2020**, *66*, 582–588. [CrossRef]
29. Diez, E.; Lopez, M.J.; Marí-Dell'Olmo, M.; Nebot, L.; Pérez, G.; Villalbi, J.R.; Carreras, R. Effects of a counselling intervention to improve contraception in deprived neighbourhoods: A randomized controlled trial. *Eur. J. Public Health* **2018**, *28*, 10–15. [CrossRef]
30. Martín, T.C. Contraceptive use patterns among Spanish single youth. *Eur. J. Contracept. Reprod. Health Care* **2005**, *10*, 219–228. [CrossRef]
31. Dueñas, J.L.; Lete, I.; Arbat, A.; Bermejo, R.; Coll, C.; Doval, J.L.; Martínez-Salmeán, J.; Pérez-Campos, E.; Serrano, I. Trends in contraception use in Spanish adolescents and young adults (15 to 24 years) between 2002 and 2008. *Eur. J. Contracept. Reprod. Health Care* **2013**, *18*, 191–198. [CrossRef]
32. Kelly, P.J.; Cheng, A.L.; Carlson, K.; Witt, J. Advanced Practice Registered Nurses and Long-Acting Reversible Contraception. *J. Midwifery Womens Health* **2017**, *62*, 190–195. [CrossRef] [PubMed]
33. Stern, L.F.; Simons, H.R.; Kohn, J.E.; Debevec, E.J.; Morfesis, J.M.; Patel, A.A. Differences in contraceptive use between family planning providers and the U.S. population: Results of a nationwide survey. *Contraception* **2015**, *91*, 464–469. [CrossRef] [PubMed]
34. Emtell Iwarsson, K.; Larsson, E.C.; Bizjak, I.; Envall, N.; Kopp Kallner, H.; Gemzell-Danielsson, K. Long-acting reversible contraception and satisfaction with structured contraceptive counselling among non-migrant, foreign-born migrant and second-generation migrant women: Evidence from a cluster randomised controlled trial (the LOWE trial) in Sweden. *BMJ Sex. Reprod. Health* **2022**, *48*, 128–136. [CrossRef] [PubMed]
35. Bastianelli, C.; Rosato, E.; Farris, M.; Benagiano, G. Emergency contraception: A survey of 1773 women. *Eur. J. Contracept. Reprod. Health Care* **2016**, *21*, 455–461. [CrossRef]
36. Bauzà, M.L.; Esteva, M.; Molina, J.; Pereiró, I.; Ingla, M.; March, S. Emergency contraception and risk habits in a university population. *Eur. J. Contracept. Reprod. Health Care* **2018**, *23*, 427–433. [CrossRef]
37. Leon-Larios, F.; Ruiz-Ferron, C.; Jalon-Neira, R.M.; Praena-Fernández, J.M. Nursing Students' Knowledge, Awareness, and Experiences of Emergency Contraception Pills' Use. *J. Clin. Med.* **2022**, *11*, 418. [CrossRef]
38. Haimovich, S. Profile of long-acting reversible contraception users in Europe. *Eur. J. Contracept. Reprod. Health Care* **2009**, *14*, 187–195. [CrossRef]
39. Sherin, M.; Waters, J. Long-acting reversible contraceptives for adolescent females: A review of current best practices. *Curr. Opin. Pediatr.* **2019**, *31*, 675–682. [CrossRef]
40. American College of Obstetricians and Gynecologists' Committee on Health Care for Underserved Women, Contraceptive Equity Expert Work Group, and Committee on Ethics. Patient-Centered Contraceptive Counseling: ACOG Committee Statement Number 1. *Obstet. Gynecol.* **2022**, *139*, 350–353. [CrossRef]
41. Paul, R.; Huysman, B.C.; Maddipati, R.; Madden, T. Familiarity and acceptability of long-acting reversible contraception and contraceptive choice. *Am. J. Obstet. Gynecol.* **2020**, *222*, S884.e1–S884.e9. [CrossRef]
42. MacCallum-Bridges, C.L.; Margerison, C.E. The Affordable Care Act contraception mandate & unintended pregnancy in women of reproductive age: An analysis of the National Survey of Family Growth, 2008–2010 vs. 2013–2015. *Contraception* **2020**, *101*, 34–39. [CrossRef] [PubMed]
43. Long, S.; Colson, L. Intrauterine Device Insertion and Removal. *Prim. Care* **2021**, *48*, 531–544. [CrossRef] [PubMed]

44. Wigginton, B.; Harris, M.L.; Loxton, D.; Lucke, J.C. A qualitative analysis of women's explanations for changing contraception: The importance of non-contraceptive effects. *J. Fam. Plan. Reprod. Health Care* **2016**, *42*, 256–262. [CrossRef] [PubMed]
45. Landersoe, S.K.; Petersen, K.B.; Vassard, D.; Larsen, E.C.; Nielsen, H.S.; Pinborg, A.; Nøhr, B.; Andersen, A.N.; Schmidt, L. Concerns on future fertility among users and past-users of combined oral contraceptives: A questionnaire survey. *Eur. J. Contracept. Reprod. Health Care* **2019**, *24*, 347–355. [CrossRef]

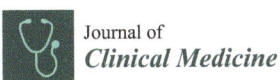

Article

Characterization of the Use of Emergency Contraception from Sentinel Pharmacies in a Region of Southern Europe

Anna M. Jambrina [1,2], Pilar Rius [3], Pilar Gascón [4], Mercè Armelles [1], Mariona Camps-Bossacoma [2], Àngels Franch [2] and Manel Rabanal [1,2,*]

1. Directorate-General for Healthcare Planning and Regulation, Ministry of Health, Government of Catalonia, 08028 Barcelona, Spain; amjambrina@gencat.cat (A.M.J.); m.armelles@gencat.cat (M.A.)
2. Physiology Section, Department of Biochemistry and Physiology, Faculty of Pharmacy and Food Science, University of Barcelona, 08028 Barcelona, Spain; marionacampsb@gmail.com (M.C.-B.); angelsfranch@ub.edu (À.F.)
3. Council of the Pharmacist's Association of Catalonia, 08009 Barcelona, Spain; prius@ccfc.cat
4. Blanquerna School of Health Sciences, Ramon Llull University, 08022 Barcelona, Spain; mariapilargl@blanquerna.url.edu
* Correspondence: mrabanal@gencat.cat

Citation: Jambrina, A.M.; Rius, P.; Gascón, P.; Armelles, M.; Camps-Bossacoma, M.; Franch, À.; Rabanal, M. Characterization of the Use of Emergency Contraception from Sentinel Pharmacies in a Region of Southern Europe. *J. Clin. Med.* **2021**, *10*, 2793. https://doi.org/10.3390/jcm10132793

Academic Editors: Francesco Maria Primiero and Giuseppe Benagiano

Received: 25 May 2021
Accepted: 22 June 2021
Published: 25 June 2021

Publisher's Note: MDPI stays neutral with regard to jurisdictional claims in published maps and institutional affiliations.

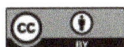

Copyright: © 2021 by the authors. Licensee MDPI, Basel, Switzerland. This article is an open access article distributed under the terms and conditions of the Creative Commons Attribution (CC BY) license (https://creativecommons.org/licenses/by/4.0/).

Abstract: Numerous studies have been published suggesting that emergency contraception (EC) is used repeatedly, but a lack of information regarding the profile of users makes it difficult to evaluate actual consumer habits. The aim of this study was to obtain information regarding the profile of users who obtain EC and other factors that might play a role, and to provide criteria to evaluate and improve the strategies of current contraceptive programs. This was an observational one-year study based on surveillance data on the provision of EC to women of reproductive age in 60 community pharmacies in Catalonia, Spain. In total, 941 notifications of dispensation of EC in Catalonia were received. A total of 44.2% of users said it was not the first time that they had taken the medication (repeat user). The percentage of users who used condoms was lower in repeat users compared to first-time users (56.7% vs. 64.4%, $p < 0.05$). A total of 25.7% of users stated that they did not use any barrier contraceptive method. The use of natural methods in repeat users was 53.8% in the subgroup who requested the medication after 48 h, significantly higher than in users who obtained the medication within the first 24 h ($p < 0.05$). A high percentage of repeat users with risky sexual behaviors were detected, suggesting that new measures must be implemented to provide information for this method, together with educational and preventive strategies.

Keywords: emergency contraception; contraceptive method; levonorgestrel; ulipristal acetate; community pharmacies; health services administration

1. Introduction

The primary aim of emergency contraception (EC) is to prevent an unwanted pregnancy following unprotected sexual intercourse. Its use has no medical contraindications and it is indicated mainly in women of reproductive age who had unprotected sex, either because they did not use contraception or the contraception failed due to inadequate or incorrect use, or because of sexual assault in which the woman was not protected by an effective contraceptive method [1–4].

The criteria for prescribing this medication are that it must not be used routinely and must never be considered a regular method of contraception, since users are not protected against sexually-transmitted diseases (STDs), including the human immunodeficiency virus (HIV) [1–4].

The medicinal products currently used in Spain as EC are post-coital pills, which contain levonorgestrel (LNG) and ulipristal acetate (UPA) as the active substances. They obtained marketing authorization in 2001 and 2009, respectively, and were initially subject to medical prescription. It was not until the end of 2009, in the case of LNG, and 2015, in the case of UPA, that they were dispensed over the counter. This allowed the population to have increased access to the medication and accorded the community pharmacist a more active role and greater responsibility in the indication and dispensing of EC [4].

For this reason, numerous practical guidelines on EC have been published in Spain since 2009, in order to ensure the rational use of the medication, guide and standardize the actions of community pharmacists to meet the demand for provision, and improve educational and preventive aspects so that users adopt safe sexual behavior [4–6].

In Europe, the World Health Organization (WHO) recommends the administration of EC as a single-dose pill that contains 1.5 mg of LNG or 30 mg of UPA. Both drugs affect the ovulation process, delaying follicular rupture, with no effects with respect to implantation of the ovum. This indicates that the efficacy of the medication decreases as time passes after unprotected intercourse. It has also been shown that, if administered after implantation of the ovum, EC is not effective at the doses indicated [1–4].

With regard to the safety of this medication, the side effects described in the product information sheets are mainly mild and transient. The most common adverse reactions are the onset of nausea and changes in the time and type of bleeding in the following menstrual period. Common adverse reactions have been reported, such as headache, myalgia, and fatigue, which typically disappear 48 h after administration of the medication. Uncommon adverse reactions identified include anorexia, ectopic pregnancy, exanthema, miscarriage, and weight gain. Multiple serious adverse events, including convulsion, ectopic pregnancy, febrile neutropenia, stroke, abdominal hernia, anaphylaxis, cancer, ovarian cyst rupture, serious infections, and suicidal ideation, have been reported [7,8].

Numerous studies have been published suggesting that this contraceptive method is used repeatedly, but a lack of information regarding the profile of users and their perception of EC as an urgent requirement makes it difficult to evaluate actual consumer habits [9]. For this reason, data that validate these suspicions need to be collected.

Currently, there are new forms of epidemiological surveillance in our setting that seek to improve the effectiveness and efficacy of detection systems and to incorporate other health indicators, such as population behavior and habits. Information on processes linked to these indicators is usually sparse or incomplete, and is typically difficult to identify with traditional surveillance tools. These processes require the integration of several agents with different professional profiles as well as having detection tools closer to the site of demand or where the event occurs. In this sense, the community pharmacist has enormous potential as a first-line agent to report the rational use of medicinal products and to educate the population to adopt safe sexual behavior [10].

In Catalonia, a region of Spain situated in South Europe, a pilot project on sentinel pharmacies, carried out in 2016, studied the dispensation of EC. The information recorded obtained the initial data on the profile of users and their patterns of behavior [11]. Nevertheless, a larger study is needed to obtain data that will allow us to develop new health indicators generated by the care dynamics of the pharmacy, reinforce traditional surveillance systems, and provide an overview of the use of this method.

Thus, the aim of this study was to obtain information regarding the profile of users who obtain EC and other factors that may be involved, and to provide criteria to evaluate and improve the strategies of current contraceptive programs.

2. Materials and Methods

This was a descriptive, observational, prospective, one-year study (July 2018–June 2019) based on surveillance data on the provision of EC in women of reproductive age (age range of 16–55 years) in community pharmacies in Catalonia, Spain, that were a part of the sentinel pharmacy network.

2.1. Sampling Frame

The Catalan sentinel pharmacy network, composed of 60 community pharmacies scattered throughout the region, was constituted proportionally to a stratification of the population of Catalonia based on criteria of representativeness, ensuring a coverage of 2.5% of the Catalan population. For the representativeness analysis, we considered the basic health areas (BHAs) of each healthcare sector of the region, establishing the proportion of urban, semi-urban, and mountain pharmacies; and considering geographical, socio-economic, demographic, epidemiological, cultural, and homogeneous communication channels.

2.2. Data Collection

Data were obtained using an 18-item electronic form that the users answered at the point of EC provision in the sentinel pharmacies. All cases were registered by 122 pharmacists from the 60 community pharmacies. The following variables were recorded:

- Code and name of sentinel pharmacy;
- Date of EC dispensation;
- National code and name of medicinal product;
- User sex (male, female);
- Age of the user;
- Who the medication is for (choice between personal use, partner, friend, daughter, and other family member);
- Postal code of the population of residence: to determine if the person searches for the medication in a nearby pharmacy;
- Time from unprotected sex (hours);
- Time since the last menstrual period (weeks);
- Contraceptive method normally used;
- First EC dispensation or not;
- If it is not the first dispensation, indicate the time elapsed since the last dispensation (less than 6 months, between 6 months and 1 year, more than 1 year);
- If it is not the first dispensation, indicate which medication was previously taken;
- If it is not the first dispensation, indicate if the patient has previously had any adverse reactions;
- Suspected adverse reactions reported to the pharmacovigilance center (yes or no);
- Description of pharmaceutical action performed;
- Availability of an EC kit consisting of a condom and additional informative material (yes or no);
- Observations (free text field to indicate any relevant aspect during the EC dispensation);

The data collection tool was validated through a pilot test carried out in 2016 in 21 community pharmacies in Barcelona, Catalonia, Spain [11].

All confidential information collected was recorded in the Applications Portal of the Ministry of Health, accessible by username and password through the Drugs and Pharmacy Channel website.

The participation rate was 99.6% (941 of 945 users). Users were informed and signed the informed consent to participate in the study.

2.3. Data Analysis

Subject characteristics that were categorical variables were summarized as counts and percentages. Continuous variables were summarized as means with standard deviations. The results related according to the type of pharmacy selected were grouped into 3 categories: urban, semi-urban, and mountain. For the statistical analysis, the χ^2 test was used for the study of the categorical variables and the Student *t*-test to compare continuous variables. A *p*-value < 0.05 was considered statistically significant. All analyses were conducted with SPSSS software, version 18 (SPSS Inc., Chicago, IL, USA).

3. Results

3.1. Incidence Data

During the study, 941 notifications of dispensation of EC in Catalonia were received (Figure 1). The months that correspond to holiday periods experienced a higher incidence in the number of dispensations; the highest were in the month of March 2019, which coincides with Easter, with an incidence of 244 per 100,000 women of reproductive age, and the summer months of August and September 2018, with an incidence of 233 per 100,000 women of reproductive age (Figure 1).

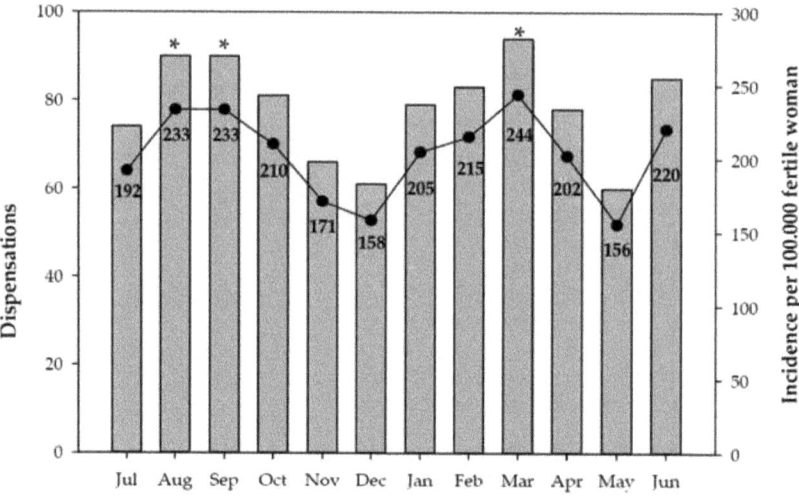

Figure 1. Number of EC dispensations and cumulative incidence per month. Catalonia, 2018–2019. Significant differences: * vs. the incidence in December ($p < 0.05$).

Similarly, urban areas reported a higher incidence in the number of dispensations with respect to semi-urban and mountain areas ($p < 0.001$ and $p < 0.05$, respectively) (Figure 2).

With respect to the type of medication, LNG was dispensed in 78.9% of cases and UPA in only 21.1%. Of all the notifications for LNG and UPA, only 12.8% and 18.6% were dispensed with an EC kit, respectively.

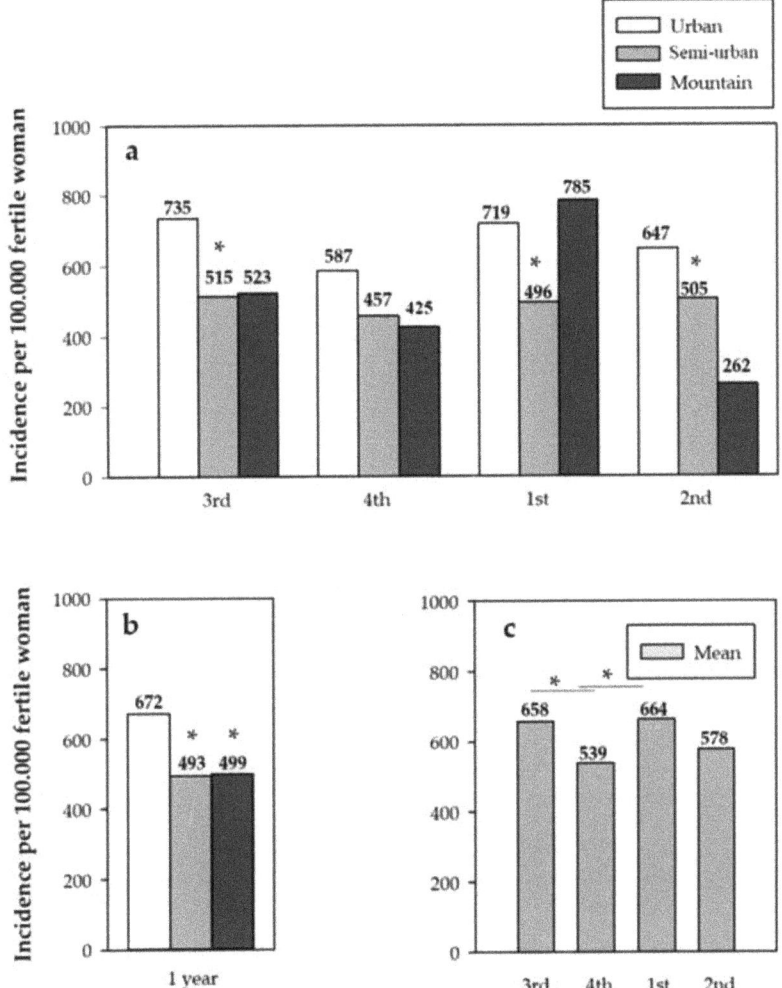

Figure 2. (a) Quarterly cumulative incidence by type of geographical area; (b) annual cumulative incidence by type of geographical area; (c) quarterly cumulative incidence in Catalonia. Significant differences: (a,b) * vs. urban area ($p < 0.05$); (c) * $p < 0.05$.

3.2. User Profile

Of the medication, 80% was dispensed to women (753 cases) and 20% was collected by men (188 cases). Almost all women (95.8%) stated that the medication was for their own use; in the case of men, 92.5% said that they collected the medication for their partner and 6.4% for a female friend. The mean age of the women was 26.9 ± 7.8 years (median of 26 years), while that of the men was 27.1 ± 9.0 years (median of 25 years), with no significant differences observed.

In relation to the patients' behavior, 55.8% of users said it was the first time that they had taken the medication (first-time user), while 44.2% stated that they had taken it on other occasions (repeat user). An increase was observed in the number of women who requested the medication when they were repeat users compared to first-time users (85.8%

vs. 75.4%, $p < 0.001$). The mean age of first-time and repeat users showed no significant differences (26.7 ± 8.4 years and 27.2 ± 7.5 years, respectively, Table 1).

Table 1. Profile of users who used EC in Catalonia during the period 2018–2019.

Variables	Total (n = 941)		Medication Collected by Women (n = 753)		Medication Collected by Men (n = 188)	
	n	%	n	%	n	%
First-time user	525	55.8	396	75.4	129	24.6
Mean age (years)	26.7 ± 8.4		26.6 ± 8.2		27.2 ± 9.1	
Condom used	338	64.4	241	60.9	97	75.2
Natural method used	129	24.6	104	26.3	25	19.4
Repeat user	416	44.2	357	85.8	59	14.2
Mean age	27.2 ± 7.5		27.3 ± 7.3		27.0 ± 8.8	
Condom used	236	56.7	201	56.3	35	59.3
Natural method used	119	28.6	99	27.7	20	33.9

Almost one-quarter of repeat users (24.3%) confirmed that they used EC less than six months previously, 23.1% used it more than six months but less than one year previously, 50.7% more than one year previously, and only 1.9% did not know this information.

Of the repeat users, 28.6% did not use any regular method of contraception compared to 24.6% of first-time users, with no significant differences observed. However, the percentage of users who used condoms was lower in the repeat users compared with first-time users (56.7% vs. 64.4%, $p < 0.05$, Table 1).

Notably, an analysis subgroup corresponded to 7.7% of cases in which the EC was dispensed to minors. In this subgroup, the medication was collected by girls in 69.4% of cases, significantly lower ($p < 0.05$) than the value for the group of repeat (85.8%) and first-time users (75.4%); mean age was 16.1 ± 1.1 years (median age of 16.5 years). Of the total number of cases, 26.4% of young people said they were repeat users; specifically, 42.1% said they had used the medication within the last six months. In general, in 31.6% of cases, young people said they did not regularly use any method of contraception, while 68.4% used condoms.

3.3. Behavior of the Users

In 87.2% of cases, the users had collected the medication within 24 h of unprotected sex; in 9.4%, in the following 25 to 48 h; and in 3.3%, after 48 h. In this regard, no statistically significant differences were observed between first-time and repeat users.

With respect to users' regular contraceptive method, the condom was the most widely used method (60.1%). However, 25.7% of users stated that they did not use any barrier contraceptive method.

Nevertheless, the joint analysis of the contraceptive methods used and risk behaviors was particularly interesting. We observed that 41.7% of the subgroup of first-time users who requested the medication between 25 and 48 h did not use any barrier method, increasing to 50% in the subgroup of first-time users who requested the medication more than 48 h after risky sexual intercourse. This was significantly higher than the proportion of first-time users who obtained the medication within 24 h of unprotected sex and who used natural methods ($p < 0.01$). Similarly, the use of natural methods in repeat users was 53.8% in the subgroup who requested the medication after 48 h, significantly higher than in users who obtained the medication within the first 24 h ($p < 0.05$) (Figure 3a).

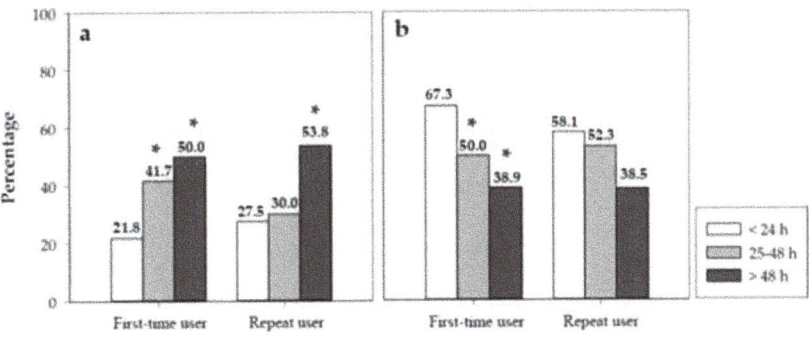

Figure 3. Percentages of first-time users and repeat users according to the time of collection of the medica-tion and their contraceptive behavior: (**a**) natural method, (**b**) preservative. Significant differ-ences: * vs. < 24 h ($p < 0.05$).

In the case of condoms, 50% and 38.9% of first-time users who collected the EC in the 25–48 h interval and after 48 h, respectively, used this contraceptive method. These percentages are significantly lower than the percentage of women who obtained the medication within the first 24 h (Figure 3b).

Likewise, when users were asked about their last menstrual period, 50% of first-time users and 30.8% of repeat users who took more than 48 h to seek EC did not remember the last time they had their period. Moreover, in 8.1% of cases, the women requested the EC more than 4 weeks after their last menstrual period.

Eighty-two percent of users said that they had obtained the EC at the pharmacy in their neighborhood (Table 2).

Table 2. Profile and behavior of users who used EC according to their area of residence.

Variables	Total		Medication Collected by Women		Medication Collected by Men	
	n	%	n	%	n	%
Same area of residence	759	82.0	607	80.0	152	20.0
Mean age (years)	26.9 ± 8.0		27.0 ± 7.7		26.7 ± 8.9	
Repeat user	332	43.7	287	86.4	45	13.5
Outside area of residence	167	18.0	135	80.8	32	19.2
Mean age (years)	26.9 ± 8.4		26.4 ± 8.1		29.1 ± 9.4	
Repeat user	77	46.1	65	84.4	12	15.6

Only 18% of cases obtained the EC in areas outside their neighborhood. No age differences were observed in the groups studied. When data from repeat users were analyzed, no differences were observed between users who obtained the medication outside their area of residence compared with the same area of residence (46.1% vs. 43.7%), while a higher percentage of women collected the medication compared to men, increasing from 80% to 86.4% in the same area of residence and to 84.4% in outside areas (Table 2).

3.4. Pharmacovigilance and Pharmaceutical Care

In relation to pharmacovigilance of the EC, 25 suspected adverse reactions were detected (2.7%), the most common being menstrual delay, dizziness, and general malaise.

In approximately half of dispensations (53.9%), the community pharmacist performed additional actions by providing the users with personalized information. The information provided included dispensing pharmacotherapeutic advice and guidance on STDs, the rational use of the medication, possible interactions with other medications, the most common side effects, problems related with the medication, and the use of alternative contraceptive methods. Furthermore, in complex cases, the pharmacist referred the patient to a gynecologist after providing advice on preventive measures and health education.

4. Discussion

Numerous studies have been conducted in recent years to determine the profile of women seeking EC, factors associated with self-reported use, and sexual behavior of users. The vast majority of these were performed using data obtained in primary care centers, hospital or primary care emergency services, and family planning clinics. In contrast, little data were obtained in community pharmacies through over-the-counter dispensing [11–13].

Contrasting the other studies, our study is one of the first carried out in the setting of a community pharmacy. Given the proximity and importance of the pharmacist as a first-line agent, we obtained a sufficiently representative sample that allowed us to characterize the population that uses EC from the care dynamic, improving knowledge of the use of this medication.

The results for the incidence of use of EC revealed that usage of this medication was higher during holiday periods: it was highest in March 2019, which coincides with Easter holidays, with an incidence of 244 per 100,000 women of reproductive age, and the summer months of August and September 2018, with an incidence of 233 per 100,000 women of reproductive age. Other national studies showed similar findings, reporting that the months in which EC was most requested were August, September, and December during the period from June 2002 to June 2004 [14].

Relevant incidence results were also obtained that show the behavioral pattern of use of EC in Catalonia, a region of Spain situated in the south of Europe. Notably, the incidence data per BHA obtained throughout the study year showed that the incidence of the use of EC is greater in urban versus rural areas. This contrasts the results obtained in a study conducted by the Catalan Ministry of Health during the period 2004 to 2007, in which a comparative analysis was performed between two geographical areas, concluding that, in the province of Lleida (rural area), the use of EC was higher than in the Barcelona metropolitan area (urban area) [15].

The results reveal the repeated use of this contraceptive method, since in 44.2% of cases users, said that it was not the first time they took this medication, which is consistent with other national and international studies [14–16].

A systematic review of the profile of EC users based on a sample of 14 articles published in Spain between 1999 and 2008 found that 9–60% of women used this medication on more than one occasion [17]. Repeat use of this medication is linked to risky sexual behavior among EC users [18,19]. In this study, the results show a higher percentage of users who do not use any regular contraceptive method and the use of condoms is lower with respect to users who take EC for the first time. Although previous studies sought to demonstrate this, the findings are inconclusive.

With respect to the age profile of the users, although we did not detect age differences between first-time and repeat users in this study, a higher overall mean age was observed in women who took EC (26.9 ± 7.8 years) in relation to data from most national and international studies, where it was 20–24 years [11,14,20,21]. However, 7.7% of EC dispensations were provided to minors, similar to that found in other studies [17]. These latter data are accompanied by a high percentage of cases that did not use any regular contraceptive method.

We observed that, in most cases, women used this medication within 24 h of having unprotected sex (87.2%), which is comparable to that obtained in other studies [14,17]. We also observed that repeat use of this medication was accompanied by more risky sexual behavior in users who take EC more than 48 h after unprotected sex compared with those who obtain it during the first few hours, including a lower percentage of users who use condoms, and a higher percentage who use no contraceptive method.

With respect to the contraceptive methods used, all studies agree that the contraceptive method most commonly used among EC users is the condom (60%), similar to the percentage in this study [14,17,20,21]. However, the percentage of users who use no contraceptive method in their sexual relationships (25.7%) is linked to a profile of users who use EC repeatedly, together with a longer time between having unprotected sex and seeking the medication, as described in other articles [14,22].

The results show a small but significant percentage of users to whom the EC was dispensed more than 4 weeks after their LMP, an aspect that requires attention and corrective measures since, according to product information sheets and therapeutic guidelines, its use after the ovulation period is not effective [1–4].

We demonstrated that there is easy access to EC, as in most cases (according to Table 2), users obtained the medication at the pharmacy in their area of residence. This also allows us to assume that the users are non-judgmental and show greater confidence with regard to healthcare professionals. Nevertheless, we found that in almost half of cases, the users who collected the medication at pharmacies outside their neighborhood used this medication repeatedly.

In addition, the Catalan sentinel pharmacy network enabled safety aspects in matters of pharmacovigilance to be reinforced by identifying suspected drug-related adverse events (DRAEs) for medicinal products marketed as EC. Fewer than 10% suspected DRAEs were reported, which is consistent with previous studies within the national setting [14]. These were mainly menstrual delay, dizziness, and general malaise, unlike other studies that reported a higher number of cases related to nausea, vomiting, and headache, described in other studies [7,8].

The demand for healthcare through low or very-low complexity processes remains mainly with pharmacies, as they are the first level of care. Accordingly, the community pharmacist has enormous potential, offering the possibility of monitoring the demand for pharmaceutical indication related with the preclinical stages of pathological processes, while having the responsibility of reporting the rational use of medicines and educating the population to adopt safe sexual behavior. Contrary to expectation, the study findings reveal low active participation of the pharmacist when dispensing the EC (53.9%), together with little medication accompanied by an EC kit. For these reasons, and as pharmaceutical care is essential for correct use of EC, more emphasis must be placed on the importance of the community pharmacist and more proactive work must be encouraged.

The main limitation of the study is that not all users were receptive to providing information at the time of dispensation of EC. However, since this occurrence was detected in the pilot test, pharmacists were trained with specific training workshops in assertive communication to address this issue [11].

Nevertheless, our study was able to show that the Catalan sentinel pharmacy network serves as a robust system for epidemiological surveillance, thus enabling data to be obtained on the profile and behavior of EC users in Catalonia. In this respect, a high percentage of repeat users was detected, with risky sexual behaviors, suggesting that new measures should be implemented to provide information on this method, together with educational and preventive strategies. It also helped to define some of the real health indicators of the general population.

Author Contributions: Conceptualization, A.M.J., À.F. and M.R.; methodology, A.M.J., P.R. and P.G.; software, M.C.-B.; validation, P.G., M.A. and À.F.; formal analysis, A.M.J. and M.C.-B.; investigation, A.M.J. and P.R.; resources, A.M.J. and P.R.; data curation, A.M.J. and M.C.-B.; writing—original draft preparation, A.M.J.; writing—review and editing, A.M.J. and P.R.; visualization, P.G. and M.A.; supervision, À.F. and M.R.; project administration, M.R.; funding acquisition, M.R. All authors have read and agreed to the published version of the manuscript.

Funding: This work was supported by the Ministry of Health, Government of Catalonia, Barcelona, Spain.

Institutional Review Board Statement: The ethical review and approval of this study was waived because no sensitive data was collected or any intervention was performed on patients.

Informed Consent Statement: Informed consent was obtained from all subjects involved in the study.

Data Availability Statement: The datasets that support the findings of this study are available from the first author (A.M.J.) upon reasonable written request.

Acknowledgments: This research was made possible by the work and dedication of the Sentinel Pharmacies Network 2017–2019 of Catalonia.

Conflicts of Interest: The authors declare no conflict of interest.

References

1. International Consortium for Emergency Contraception (ICEC); International Federation of Gynecology and Obstetrics (FIGO). *Emergency Contraceptive Pills: Medical and Service Delivery Guidance*, 4th ed.; International Consortium for Emergency Contraception: New York, NY, USA, 2018. Available online: https://www.cecinfo.org/wp-content/uploads/2018/12/ICEC-guides_FINAL.pdf (accessed on 3 March 2021).
2. World Health Organization. *WHO Organization Selected Practice Recommendations for Contraceptive Use*, 3rd ed.; World Health Organization: Geneva, Switzerland, 2016; Available online: https://apps.who.int/iris/handle/10665/252267 (accessed on 3 March 2021).
3. World Health Organization. *WHO Medical Eligibility Criteria for Contraceptive Use*, 5th ed.; World Helath Organization: Geneva, Switzerland, 2015. Available online: https://apps.who.int/iris/handle/10665/181468 (accessed on 12 March 2021).
4. European Consortium for Emergency Contraception; ECEC Emergency Contraception. *A Guideline for Service Provision in Europe*, 2nd ed.; European Consortium for Emergency Contraception: Tirgu Mores, Romania, 2016. Available online: http://www.smicontraccezione.it/documenti/ecec-lg-europa-2016.pdf (accessed on 12 March 2021).
5. Ministry of Health of Spain. Clinical Practice Guideline for Hormonal and Intrauterine Contraception. 2019. Available online: https://portal.guiasalud.es/wp-content/uploads/2019/06/gpc_585_anticoncepcion_iacs_compl.pdf (accessed on 12 March 2021).
6. Spanish Society of Contraception. Emergency Contraception Protocol. 2019. Available online: https://www.ec-ec.org/wp-content/uploads/2020/02/SEC-2019-Guia-AU-.pdf (accessed on 15 March 2021).
7. Leelakanok, N.; Methaneethorn, J. A systematic review and meta-analysis of the adverse effects of levonorgestrel emergency oral contraceptive. *Clin. Drug Investig.* **2020**, *40*, 395–420. [CrossRef] [PubMed]
8. Jatlaoui, T.C.; Riley, H.; Curtis, K.M. Safety data for levonorgestrel, ulipristal acetate and Yuzpe regimens for emergency contraception. *Contraception* **2016**, *93*, 93–112. [CrossRef] [PubMed]
9. Halpern, V.; Raymond, E.G.; Lopez, L.M. Repeated use of pre- and postcoital hormonal contraception for prevention of pregnancy. *Cochrane Database Syst. Rev.* **2014**, *26*, CD007595. Available online: https://www.cochranelibrary.com/cdsr/doi/10.1002/14651858.CD007595.pub3/full (accessed on 30 March 2021). [CrossRef] [PubMed]
10. Gonsalves, L.; Hindin, M.J. Pharmacy provision of sexual and reproductive health commodities to young people: A systematic literature review and synthesis of the evidence. *Contraception* **2017**, *95*, 339–363. [CrossRef] [PubMed]
11. Jambrina, A.M.; Rabanal, M.; Guayta, R.; Rius, P.; Gascón, P.; Rodríguez, G.; Fernández, R.; Davins, J.; Rams, N.; Gaspar, M.J. Pilot program of sentinel pharmacies. Follow-up of the dispensing of emergency contraception in Catalonia during 2016. *Butlletí Epidemiològic Catalunya* **2016**, *37*, 278–284.
12. Uysal, J.; Tavrow, P.; Hsu, R.; Alterman, A. Availability and accessibility of emergency contraception to adolescent callers in pharmacies in four Southwestern States. *J. Adolesc. Health* **2018**, *64*, 219–225. [CrossRef] [PubMed]
13. Wilkinson, T.A.; Rafie, S.; Clark, P.D.; Carroll, A.E.; Miller, E. Evaluating community pharmacy responses about levonorgestrel emergency contraception by mystery caller characteristics. *J. Adolesc. Health* **2018**, *63*, 32–36. [CrossRef] [PubMed]
14. Santamaría, T.; Crespo, A.V.; Cid, A.; Gontán, M.J.; González, M.; Baz, C.; Sánchez, R. Emergency contraceptive: Profile of the users and demand characteristics. *SEMERGEN* **2006**, *32*, 321–324.
15. Ros, C.; Miret, M.; Rué, M. Descriptive study of the use of emergency contraception in Catalonia (Spain): Comparison between a rural and an urban area. *Gac. Sanit.* **2009**, *23*, 496–500. [CrossRef] [PubMed]
16. Serra-Torres, A.; Montaner-Amorós, M.; Sitjar-Martínez de Sas, S.; Sisó-Almirall, A.; Espanyol-Navarro, M.; Devant-Altimir, M. Emergency Contraception: Evaluation of Women's Understanding of It, a Requisite for the Effectiveness of the Treatment. *Atención Primaria* **2007**, *39*, 87–91. [CrossRef] [PubMed]
17. Bauzà, M.L.; Esteva, M.; Pereiro, I.; Ingla, M. Systematic Review of the profile of emergency contraception users. *Rev. Latino-Am. Enfermagem.* **2016**, *24*, e2733. [CrossRef]
18. Girma, S.; Paton, D. The impact of emergency birth control on teen pregnancy and STIs. *J. Health Econ.* **2011**, *30*, 373–380. [CrossRef] [PubMed]
19. Tydén, T.; Palmqvist, M.; Larsson, M. A repeated survey of sexual behaviour among female university students in Sweden. *Acta Obstet. Gynecol. Scand.* **2012**, *91*, 215–219. [CrossRef] [PubMed]

20. Soon, J.A.; Levine, M.; Osmond, B.L.; Ensom, M.H.; Fielding, D.W. Effects of making emergency contraception available without a physician's prescription: A population-based study. *CMAJ* **2005**, *29*, 878–883. [CrossRef] [PubMed]
21. Marston, C.; Meltzer, H.; Majeed, A. Impact on contraceptive practice of making emergency hormonal contraception available over the counter in Great Britain: Repeated cross sectional surveys. *BMJ* **2005**, *331*, 271–275. [CrossRef] [PubMed]
22. Vergara, J.C.; López-Guerrero, A.; López, F. Emergency Contraception: Users Profile in Primary Care Emergency Services. *Atención Primaria* **2004**, *34*, 279–285.

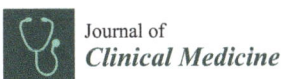

Article

Nursing Students' Knowledge, Awareness, and Experiences of Emergency Contraception Pills' Use

Fatima Leon-Larios [1], Cecilia Ruiz-Ferron [1,2,*], Rocio-Marina Jalon-Neira [3] and Juan-Manuel Praena-Fernández [1,4]

1. Nursing Department, Faculty of Nursing, Physiotherapy and Podiatry, University of Seville, 41009 Seville, Spain; fatimaleon@us.es (F.L.-L.); jpraena_2@ugr.es (J.-M.P.-F.)
2. University Hospital Virgen del Rocío, 41013 Seville, Spain
3. Aljarafe District, Health Andalusian Service, 41917 Seville, Spain; marina_jalon@hotmail.com
4. Unit Biostatistic, Department of Statistics, Faculty of Medicine, University of Granada, 18016 Granada, Spain
* Correspondence: mruiz8@us.es

Abstract: The emergency contraception pill (ECP) is a non-prescribed medication in Spain. However, there is not enough evidence of its use among young people to define sex education contents. The aims of this research were to describe the experiences of the use of the ECP in university students and analyze their knowledge, attitude, and awareness regarding the ECP. The cross-sectional, analytic study was conducted with nursing degree students at the University of Seville. A total of 478 students answered the questionnaire. All of the students (100%) had heard about the ECP and had a positive attitude towards this contraceptive. A total of 25.7% had used the ECP, mainly because a condom had failed or because they did not use any contraceptive at all. Deficiencies in knowledge are related with the ECPs' mechanism of action, efficacy after repeated use, and the type of ECP available. Female students who used no method at all or withdrawal, and who were over 20 years old, used ECP to a greater extent ($p < 0.005$). Further education initiatives focused on the use of the ECP, its efficacy, and typology are needed, particularly among future health professionals who will later educate other young people.

Keywords: emergency contraception pills; morning-after pill; levonorgestrel; ulipristal acetate; sexual behavior; students; contraceptive knowledge; contraceptive attitude; contraceptive experience

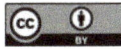

1. Introduction

Emergency contraception (EC) is used to prevent pregnancy if the chosen contraceptive has failed or if no contraception was used. Under no circumstances must it be considered a contraception method to be used on a regular basis. The use of an emergency contraception pill (ECP) is recommended as soon as possible whenever sexual intercourse with a chance of pregnancy has occurred, preferably within the first 12 h postcoitum, the first 72 h if levonorgestrel (LNG) is administered, or within the first 5 days when using ulipristal acetate (UPA). The mechanism of action of EC is avoiding pregnancy, inhibiting or delaying ovulation, but not preventing implantation of a fertilized egg. This drug will neither cause an abortion nor embryo damage [1]. However, it must be taken into account that this drug does not offer any protection against sexually transmitted infections (STI) [2,3].

The distribution of the ECP in Spain has changed in the last years; it can be administered in pharmacies without prescription, since 2009 for LNG and since 2015 for UPA [4]. This facilitates access to young people [3], though the vulnerable population may face difficulties in this access as the dispensation cost of this drug must be borne by the user [5]. The fact that access and purchase are easy means that young people must have information on its usage, effects, and management [6]. Despite its common use, around 30–50% of young people under the age of 30 have used the ECP at some point in their lives, knowledge about this drug is scarce [7–10]. The use pattern is related to its availability and accessibility in combination with individual knowledge and awareness of ECP [9,11].

Sex education training nowadays has proved to be poor [12–14], and in many cases it does not include information on the ECP. Sexual education has been proven to impact sexual behavior, the latter becoming healthier [15,16]. Even in the setting of university stages, sex education in contraception and sexual health is needed, particularly for health professionals who can include sex education in their teaching activities [17,18]. Notwithstanding this, it has been observed that in studies related to Health Science, students develop healthier behaviors and acquire more knowledge in this field than those students pursuing their degrees in other fields [13].

The objectives of this study were basically three: (1) describe the experiences of ECP users at university stages; (2) analyze their knowledge on ECP; (3) define both attitudes and awareness around ECP with the aim of designing educational programs at university level.

2. Materials and Methods

2.1. Study Design

A cross-sectional, analytic, descriptive study was carried out. Participants were male and female students of the nursing degree during the academic years 2019–20 and 2020–21 at Universidad de Sevilla. Male students were asked about their experience with their partners regarding ECP use. The questionnaire was performed prior to the seminar on family planning programmed for the subject Nursing in Reproductive Health, which includes content related to ECP use. The aim was to identify any lack of knowledge, level of awareness, plus attitudes and experiences regarding the ECP.

2.2. Measures

The questionnaire administered online was created ad hoc based on the existing literature [8,19–23] by the first two authors and agreed by the four authors. Socio-demographic variables of sex, age, and sexual orientation were included. Students were asked about their sexual behavior, ECP use and reasons to use it, time gap after sexual intercourse and use, ECP use recommendations to others, symptomatology associated with ECP use, and if they felt embarrassed when they purchased it at the pharmacy.

Moreover, students were asked about their knowledge of the ECP (10 questions posed in affirmative and negative forms that could be answered with true, false, do not know/no answer) and its mechanism of action and effects. Each correct answer scored 1 point, and each wrong answer or no answer added 0 points, each participant obtained a mark out of a total score of 10 points.

2.3. Data Collection

Data regarding the period October 2019–October 2020 were collected through an online questionnaire via Google Drive. This questionnaire was pilot tested by 10 students in order to identify potential weaknesses. Once the review process ended, the final version was launched. Students were provided with a link to a questionnaire form to be completed from their mobile devices (phone or laptop).

2.4. Ethical Aspects

Anonymity and confidentiality when answering the questionnaire was granted at all times. Prior to the completion of the questionnaire, students were informed about the objectives of the study and they also were asked for their consent to participate with their data in the study. All the information was provided by the students. Ethical review and approval were waived due to the research being an anonymous web-based study, thus it did not require approval.

2.5. Data Analysis

An exploratory data analysis was performed in order to identify any possible outliers. This analysis took into account the whole population studied, as well as the different subgroups created. An exploratory graph analysis of the different studied variables according to their numeric or non-numeric character was conducted. Frequency distribution and percentages were used for the descriptive analysis of qualitative (non-numeric) variables. For quantitative (numeric) variables, centrality and dispersion statistics were calculated.

The relation between two qualitative variables was analyzed through Pearson's chi-square test, Yates's chi-square test, linear-by-linear association test, and Fisher's exact test, according to mandatory criteria. Significant results of these tests were completed with a 95% confidence interval (CI) for percentage differences.

With respect to numeric variables between two groups, the Student's t-test was applied to compare the means, the requirements of normality and randomness were validated (Kolmogorov–Smirnov test or Shapiro–Wilks test according to sample size) and the F-test was used for equality of variances (Levene's test). When the latter did not work, the Student's T-test was performed for independent samples with Welch's correction. When normality requirements were not met, the Mann–Whitney U test was applied.

For the comparison of numeric variables between more than two groups, and once the requirements of independence, normality, and homoscedasticity were validated, the ANOVA test (Analysis of variance) was applied. When requirements were not met, the Kruskal–Wallis test was applied. In order to determine the risk factors associated with EC use, a logistic regression model was applied obtaining both the crude and adjusted odds ratio at a 95% confidence interval.

In all hypothesis contrasts, the significance level was set at 0.05. Data analysis was processed by IBM SPSS 26 (IBM Corp., Armonk, NY, USA).

3. Results

A total of 478 students took part in the study during the academic years 2019/20 and 2020/21. All participants accepted to answer the questionnaire in the first 10–15 min of the workshop where they were going to receive information about contraception as part of the curricula of the nursing degree, so the rate of response was 100%. No student refused to participate.

The majority of participants were under the age of 25, with an average age of 20.87 (SD 4.52). Participants' socio-demographic variables are indicated in Table 1, as well as sexual behaviors, and sex-disaggregated contraceptive use.

Table 1. Socio-demographic characteristics.

Socio-Demographic Variables	Total % (n) 100 (478)	Men [1] % (n) 18.8 (90)	Women % (n) 81.2 (288)	p-Value
Age (years), Mean (SD)	20.87 (4.52)	22.13 (6.48)	20.58 (3.88)	0.003
Sexual orientation, % (n)				
Heterosexual	86.2 (412)	84.3 (75)	87.1 (337)	
Homosexual	3.1 (15)	10.1 (9)	1.6 (6)	n.a. [2]
Bisexual	10.3 (49)	5.6 (5)	11.4 (44)	
Have you had any intercourse? Yes, % (n)	83.9 (401)	93.3 (84)	81.7 (317)	0.006
Age of first sexual intercourse, Median (SD)	16.53 (1.46)	16.99 (1.57)	16.41 (1.41)	0.001
Received any information on the ECP, Yes, % (n)	70.5 (337)	74.4 (67)	69.6 (270)	0.442

[1] Male students answered question in relation to their sexual partners. [2] Not applicable.

The average age for first sexual encounters was 16.53 (1.46), differentiating males (16.99 ± 1.57 years) and females (16.41 ± 1.46) years, $p < 0.001$, (IC 0.225–0.924). Male students declared themselves more sexually active than their female peers, 83.9% of participants allegedly having any kind of sexual intercourse. In opposition to national statistics, in this sample, male students proved to have their first sexual encounter later than girls.

Participants were asked for the contraceptive methods used throughout their sex life. The most common contraceptive method is the condom (77.4% (370)), followed by hormonal methods (pill, patch, and ring) (32.8% (157)). A high percentage of young people still use coitus interruptus as a method to avoid pregnancy (27% (129)), and almost 7.9% (38) do not use any method during their sexual relations as shown in Figure 1.

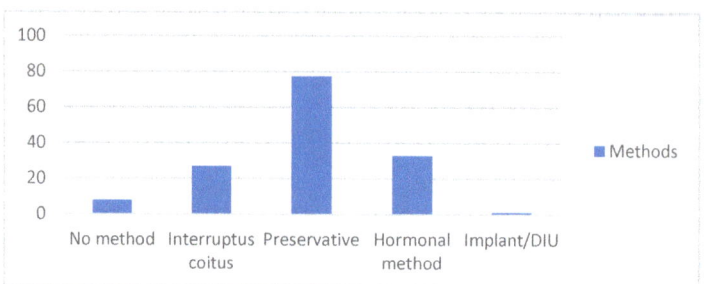

Figure 1. Contraceptive methods used at some point of the sex life (%).

In total, 7 out of 10 students declared they had been provided with some type of information on contraception methods, including the emergency contraceptive pill. The major information sources of those who acknowledged having received previous training were via health professionals (48.96% (165)), the Internet (32.34% (109)), and at school (25.51% (86)), as shown in Figure 2.

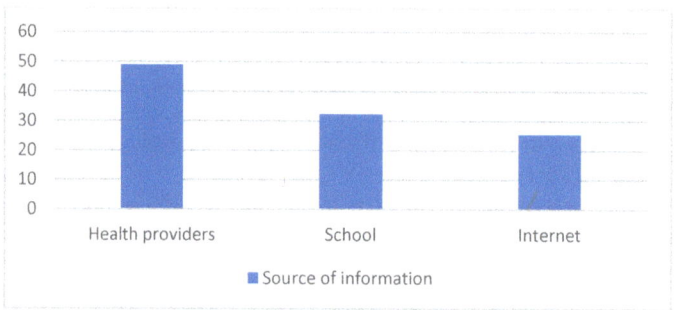

Figure 2. Previous education on contraceptive methods.

3.1. ECP Use and Attitudes

In all, 100% of participants showed awareness about ECP. A total of 25.7% (123) had used the ECP: 69.1% (85) of these just once, 19.5% (24) two times, 10.6% (13) three times, and 0.8% (1) up to five times. There were some significant differences ($p < 0.001$) between female (34.7%) and male students (15.5%).

The main reason indicated for using the ECP was due to any issue regarding the condom (it broke or came off) (3.41%, 78 participants), 37.77% (44) did not use any method consistently during sexual intercourse or tried ineffectually a withdrawal/coitus interruptus. After using the ECP, 33.3% (41) changed to another contraceptive method. A total of 33.3% (41) of ECP users had after effects after the use of the ECP, the most common being nausea/vomiting (34.78% (16)), irregular bleeding (28.26% (13)), general unrest (23.91% (11)), and headache (13.04 (6)). Despite female students suffering from these symptoms, a total of 58.5% (24) would recommend its use to other women if they needed it. In general terms, 80.5% (99) of participants using the ECP did not recall which type of pill it was, and 77.2% (95) used it within the first 12 h, regardless the student's sex or age ($p = 0.72$).

Female participants who used the ECP had their first sexual intercourse at a younger age (15.76 (1.31)) than those who did not (16.87 (1.40)), which was statistically significant ($p < 0.001$). In total, 82.9% (102) had a steady partner when they used the ECP, and 62.6% (77)

felt embarrassed when they had to purchase it at the pharmacy. Approximately two-thirds (66.7% (82)) of participants who used it would recommend it use to others, with similar results among female and male students. There is no relation between having received previous information on the ECP and its use: 27.1% did not receive any information and 32% did ($p = 0.392$).

More than half of the participants (58.6% (280)) considered that the ECP should be free, with no significant differences in sex or opinion among people who had used them and those who did not ($p = 0.12$). Only three students (2.4%) in the sample had undergone a voluntary termination of pregnancy, and all of them had used the ECP at some point in their lives. One of these students had used the ECP once; the other two, more than once. The age of their first sexual encounter was below the sample mean.

3.2. Knowledge about ECP

Questions about the ECP are indicated in Table 2, the students' answers segregated by sex. Percentage of success is indicated. It is observed that 4 out of 10 men thought that the ECP mechanism of action is abortion, and 5 out of 10 men considered the ECP a contraceptive method. Almost half of the female and male students considered that the ECP may harm the embryo if the woman is pregnant.

Table 2. Knowledge about ECP by sex.

Item	Men	Women	p-Value
	Correct (n)%	Correct (n)%	
1. ECP are abortive, lead to embryo abortion, False	58.9 (53)	75.5 (293)	0.001
2. A medical prescription is needed to purchase the postcoital pill, False	82.2 (74)	87.9 (341)	0.167
3. If the woman is pregnant, the pill may harm the zygote or embryo, False	48.9 (44)	46.6 (181)	0.726
4. The ECP protect against sexual transmission infections (STI), False	100 (90)	98.2 (381)	0.357
5. There is one type of oral emergency contraception that can be used within 5 days after risk of pregnancy sex, True	38.9 (35)	35.3 (137)	0.543
6. Morning-after pill affects women's reproductive health in the long term, reducing the possibilities to conceive on later life stages, False	50 (45)	49.7 (193)	1.000
7. Efficacy of postcoital contraception is reduced each hour after risk of pregnancy sex, True	75.6 (68)	78.4 (304)	0.575
8. A pregnancy test is required prior to take ECP, False	83.3 (75)	86.1 (334)	0.507
9. Postcoital pills can be used whenever necessary, without affecting its efficacy, True	5.6 (5)	6.7 (26)	0.816
10. ECP is a contraceptive method, False	50 (45)	66.8 (259)	0.004

The use of ulipristal acetate as an oral emergency contraceptive within the first 5 days after the risk of pregnancy was known by 5 out of 10 students. There was an erroneous belief that ECPs reduce their effect with repeated use.

Most participants were aware of the fact that the use of ECPs does not protect from STIs, and knew that neither a medical prescription nor a pregnancy test are needed for its use. Between 7–8 of 10 students were aware that the time after sexual intercourse is crucial for the efficacy of the ECP.

There is no relation between the age when the first sexual encounter takes place and the score obtained in the test ($p = 0.069$). However, the students ranking higher in the questionnaire were those who had received previous information in the subject, 6.42 vs. 5.81 over 10 scores ($p < 0.001$). Likewise, female students who had received any kind of sex education on this aspect obtained higher scores (6.51 vs. 5.86, $p < 0.001$), while male students' answers show no statistically significant differences (6.06 vs. 5.57, $p = 0.209$).

Students who had used the ECP obtained higher scores in the knowledge test (6.61 ± 1.56 vs. 6.13 ± 1.68), $p = 0.007$). The level of knowledge regarding each item does not condition the recommendation of the use of the ECP to females that may need it ($p > 0.05$).

Table 3 illustrates the factors independently associated to ECP use are age (20 years old), sex (woman), contraceptive method used, and knowledge about ECP. These factors jointly maintain the risk of significant use.

Table 3. Risk factors associated to ECP use.

	Crude OR (95% CI)	p-Value	Adjusted OR (95% CI)	p-Value
Age * (older than 20 years)	3.08 (1.98; 4.79)	<0.001	3.04 (1.92; 4.79)	<0.001
Sex (Woman)	2.90 (1.53; 5.47)	0.001	2.87 (1.47; 5.61)	0.002
Had you ever received any information/guidance on postcoital contraception? (Yes)	1.26 (0.77; 2.06)	0.35		
Contraceptive Methods ** (Withdrawal/No method)	2.02 (1.31; 3.12)	0.001	1.90 (1.20; 3.01)	0.006
Total score	1.19 (1.05; 1.37)	0.008	1.16 (1.01; 1.34)	0.032

* Age variable was stacked in younger and older than 20 years old. ** Contraceptive methods variable was stacked in users of consistent contraceptive use and users of withdrawal/no method at all.

4. Discussion

The aim of this study was to explore the knowledge, attitudes, awareness, and experiences of university students of the nursing degree at the Universidad de Sevilla regarding ECP, in order to define the educational action needed as future health agents educating young people in this matter.

An increased use of the ECP was expected with the arrival of deregulated access to ECPs in pharmacies. However, it has been observed that there had only been a slight increase that had disappeared over the years [24] or the use had remained stable [8]. Results of this study revealed that the totality of the students had heard about EC, as also observed in other studies [25]. The prevalence of drug use in this sample (25.7%) is similar to other published studies with Spanish cohorts [12,17], and those from other countries [10,26]; however, this prevalence is lower than that observed in other studies [19,27]. Almost all participants were knowledgeable about the fact that the ECP required no medical prescription for its purchase and use; other studies with university students showing similar results [26,28].

Access to ECPs is more difficult when people lack the knowledge or the socioeconomic resources [5,29]. All participants in the sample were university students and maybe this fact could be the reason for a higher prevalence of use [8,9] with respect to other disadvantaged groups. Both the ECP access price (around EUR 20) and knowledge as to how to access it may condition its use [8,24]. More than half of the participants considered that ECPs should be free, with no significant difference in opinion between the students' sex. The most common type of ECP used was levonorgestrel, as also indicated in other studies conducted in other countries [30–32], despite it being proved that UPA is more effective in preventing pregnancy [33]. Our results showed that participants were not aware of the existence of an ECP that is effective up to 5 days after the risk of pregnancy sex, with the mechanism of action of an ECP.

It was observed that those students having sexual intercourse at an earlier age had used EC in a larger proportion than those who had delayed their first sexual experience. This could be due to higher sexual risk behavior at earlier ages [19,21,34]. The onset of sexual intercourse of the sample is consistent with the average Spanish youth [13].

In line with results obtained by Jiménez-Iglesias, users of the ECP in this study did not change their usual contraceptive method after ECP use [12]. As other studies with young people have proved, condoms are the most commonly used contraceptive method, and the main cause of EC use is the condom breaking/slipping or not using any contraception method at all [7,21,30,34,35], showing similar results to this study with university students. In the light of the results obtained, and the high percentage of users who declared to have experienced a condom break/slip, it is necessary to reinforce education on the correct use of this contraceptive method in order to avoid this recurrence. Moreover, it is necessary to place particular emphasis on the fact that coitus interruptus is not a contraceptive method to prevent unintended pregnancy.

Studies conducted in the United Kingdom and the USA on the contraceptive consumption profile showed that it was more used among single women [9,17,36] than among those who had a partner, those who had had an abortion in the last 5 years [8], and those women who used less consistent contraceptives [8,24]. However, this study shows how most participants had a partner when they used EC and were using a condom as a contraceptive method during sexual intercourse [4]. Only three participants had undergone a voluntary abortion procedure, and all of them had used the ECP at least once and had early sexual relationships compared to the average.

As shown in previous studies, the use of EC took place within the first 24 h after unprotected sexual intercourse [4], and mainly within the first 12 h, with no differences observed regarding the student's age [30]. Three out of ten women declared to have taken the ECP more than once, similar to results obtained in other European countries [31,37], and this shows the need for reinforcing the information provided about the correct use of contraceptive methods and thus avoiding repeated use of EC.

It has been observed that awareness, attitudes, and beliefs influence contraceptive use [38]. As shown in similar researches, though awareness of EC is ample, the students' knowledge on EC can be improved [20,22,27,39]. In particular, the extended beliefs on its efficacy, side effects, and attitudes towards ECP, condition its use [8,10]. In our study, we observed the erroneous beliefs regarding the ECP's mechanism of action, a question already identified in other studies with nursing students [40]. The belief that EC intake affects women's fertility in the future has been revealed in previous studies [17,22], and it is in line with our results, as only half of the participants knew that the use of the ECP does not necessarily affect women's fertility or have consequences in the long term due to repeated use [2,41,42]. There is no evidence of efficacy loss due to repeated use, but this erroneous belief seems widely spread among participants [17]. Though some studies point to the fact that young women are better informed about EC [7], this study cannot confirm this evidence, in light of the results obtained [43].

There is a correlation between having received previous information on ECP and its use [8], a result in accordance with the findings of this study. Moreover, this information was more effective among young women, who showed better knowledge [39], but our study found no difference between male and female students regarding their knowledge on EC, both groups obtaining very similar scoring. The major sources of information were health professionals and the Internet, while other studies indicated the school [44], Internet [45], or friends [22] were major information sources.

In this study, male students were asked about their knowledge, attitudes, and experiences regarding EC, taking as a reference their sexual partner as the one who took the ECP. The study conducted by Richards et al. (2016) already revealed that young men wanted to be involved in the decision making regarding contraception in their relationships, and also showed interest in knowing more about EC [46]. This fact is confirmed in this study, where they actively participated with their answers and showed a similar knowledge level to that of their female peers in almost all items. It is therefore necessary to foster and encourage their participation in all formative initiatives aimed at the youth.

Limitations

This study was conducted using a sample of university students in southern Spain, and, thus, similar results cannot be expected for other knowledge areas or other regions in the country. As students related to health sciences, it is possible to conclude that they may be more knowledgeable and possess a healthier attitude towards this subject [13,47] than those students focusing in other studies. Furthermore, the absence of cultural diversity in the sample does not allow exploration of this aspect. Due to the cross-sectional nature of the study, causality cannot be proved.

5. Conclusions

All university students showed an awareness about EC and, in general, a positive attitude towards its use. One out of three university students who used the ECP, showed a lack of knowledge regarding its mechanisms of action, efficacy, and the types of ECP. This study helps to define the formative contents regarding the ECP aimed at university students in order to ensure their sex education and information on emergency contraception is adequate. It is necessary to address the issues detected both as users and health professionals who will advise others in the future, so that the information they provide is based on scientific evidence.

Author Contributions: Conceptualization, F.L.-L. and C.R.-F.; methodology, J.-M.P.-F., F.L.-L. and C.R.-F.; formal analysis, F.L.-L. and J.-M.P.-F.; investigation, writing—original draft preparation, F.L.-L., J.-M.P.-F., C.R.-F. and R.-M.J.-N.; writing—review and editing, F.L.-L., J.-M.P.-F., C.R.-F. and R.-M.J.-N. All authors have read and agreed to the published version of the manuscript.

Funding: This research received no external funding.

Institutional Review Board Statement: The study was conducted according to the guidelines of the Declaration of Helsinki. Ethical review and approval were waived for this study due to students being invited to participate voluntarily.

Informed Consent Statement: Informed consent was obtained from all subjects involved in the study.

Data Availability Statement: All data generated or analyzed during this study are included in this published article.

Conflicts of Interest: The authors declare no conflict of interest.

References

1. FIGO. Mechanism of Action for Emergency Contraception I FIGO. 2021. Available online: https://www.figo.org/mechanism-action-emergency-contraception (accessed on 22 November 2021).
2. Leelakanok, N.; Methaneethorn, J. A Systematic Review and Meta-analysis of the Adverse Effects of Levonorgestrel Emergency Oral Contraceptive. *Clin. Drug Investig.* **2020**, *40*, 395–420. [CrossRef] [PubMed]
3. Raine, T.R.; Harper, C.C.; Rocca, C.H.; Fischer, R.; Padian, N.; Klausner, J.D.; Darney, P.D. Direct access to emergency contraception through pharmacies and effect on unintended pregnancy and STIs: A randomized controlled trial. *JAMA* **2005**, *293*, 54–62. [CrossRef]
4. Jambrina, A.M.; Rius, P.; Gascón, P.; Armelles, M.; Camps-Bossacoma, M.; Franch, À.; Rabanal, M. Characterization of the Use of Emergency Contraception from Sentinel Pharmacies in a Region of Southern Europe. *J. Clin. Med.* **2021**, *10*, 2793. [CrossRef] [PubMed]
5. Barbosa, R.M.; Kalckmann, S.; Arilha, M.; Giacomo do Lago, T.D. The emergency contraceptive pill in Brazil: High usage rates but schooling differences persist. *Contraception* **2021**, *104*, 401–405. [CrossRef] [PubMed]
6. Hussain, R.; Kavanaugh, M.L. Changes in use of emergency contraceptive pills in the United States from 2008 to 2015. *Contraception* **2021**, *10*, 100065. [CrossRef]
7. Bauzà, M.L.; Esteva, M.; Molina, J.; Pereiró, I.; Ingla, M.; March, S. Emergency contraception and risk habits in a university population. *Eur. J. Contracept. Reprod. Health Care* **2018**, *23*, 427–433. [CrossRef] [PubMed]

8. Heller, C.; Perreira, K.M.; Shartzer, A.; Johnston, E.M.; Courtot, B. Emergency Contraception Use: The Influence of Awareness, Attitudes, and Beliefs among Non-Hispanic White, Non-Hispanic Black, and Hispanic Women in the United States. *Women's Health Issues* **2019**, *29*, 161–169. [CrossRef]
9. Chofakian, C.B.; Moreau, C.; Borges, A.L.V.; Dos Santos, O.A. Contraceptive discontinuation: Frequency and associated factors among undergraduate women in Brazil. *Reprod. Health* **2019**, *16*, 131. [CrossRef] [PubMed]
10. Nappi, R.E.; Lobo Abascal, P.; Mansour, D.; Rabe, T.; Shojai, R. Emergency Contraception Study Group. Use of and attitudes towards emergency contraception: A survey of women in five European countries. *Eur. J. Contracept. Reprod. Health Care* **2014**, *19*, 93–101. [CrossRef]
11. Williams, B.N.; Jauk, V.C.; Szychowski, J.M.; Arbuckle, J.L. Adolescent emergency contraception usage, knowledge, and perception. *Contraception* **2021**, *103*, 361–366. [CrossRef]
12. Jiménez-Iglesias, A.; Moreno, C.; García-Moya, I.; Rivera, F. Prevalence of emergency contraceptive pill use among Spanish adolescent girls and their family and psychological profiles. *BMC Women's Health* **2018**, *18*, 67. [CrossRef]
13. Leon-Larios, F.; Macías-Seda, J. Factors related to healthy sexual and contraceptive behaviors in undergraduate students at university of Seville: A cross-sectional study. *Reprod. Health* **2017**, *14*, 179. [CrossRef]
14. Martínez, J.L.; Vicario-Molina, I.; González, E.; Ilabaca, P. Sex education in Spain: The relevance of teachers' training and attitudes/Educación sexual en España: Importancia de la formación y las actitudes del profesorado. *J. Study Educ. Dev.* **2014**, *37*, 117–148. [CrossRef]
15. Morales, A.; Espada, J.P.; Orgilés, M. A 1-year follow-up evaluation of a sexual-health education program for Spanish adolescents compared with a well-established program. *Eur. J. Public Health* **2016**, *26*, 35–41. [CrossRef]
16. Morales, A.; Orgilés, M.; Espada, J.P. Sexually Unexperienced Adolescents Benefit the Most From a Sexual Education Program for Adolescents: A Longitudinal Cluster Randomized Controlled Study. *AIDS Educ. Prev.* **2020**, *32*, 493–511. [CrossRef]
17. Amengual, M.L.; Canto, M.E.; Berenguer, I.P.; Pol, M.I. Systematic Review of the profile of emergency contraception users. *Rev. Lat. Am. Enfermagem* **2016**, *24*, e2733. [CrossRef] [PubMed]
18. Sharon, D.; Gonen, A.; Linetsky, I. Factors influencing nursing students' intention to practice sexuality education in their professional work. *Am. J. Sex. Educ.* **2020**, *15*, 262–278. [CrossRef]
19. Abera, L.; Sema, A.; Guta, A.; Belay, Y. Emergency contraceptive utilization and associated factors among college students in Dire Dawa City, Eastern Ethiopia: A cross-sectional study. *Eur. J. Midwifery* **2021**, *5*, 28. [CrossRef] [PubMed]
20. Addo, V.N.; Tagoe-Darko, E.D. Knowledge, practices, and attitudes regarding emergency contraception among students at a university in Ghana. *Int. J. Gynaecol. Obstet.* **2009**, *105*, 206–209. [CrossRef]
21. Bauzà-Amengual, M.L.; Esteva, M.; Ingla-Pol, M.; Font-Oliver, M.A.; March, S. Discourses on the postcoital pill in young women. *BMC Public Health* **2018**, *18*, 803. [CrossRef] [PubMed]
22. Asut, O.; Ozenli, O.; Gur, G.; Deliceo, E.; Cagin, B.; Korun, O.; Turk, O.; Vaizoglu, S.; Cali, S. The knowledge and perceptions of the first year medical students of an International University on family planning and emergency contraception in Nicosia (TRNC). *BMC Women's Health* **2018**, *18*, 149. [CrossRef]
23. Hoque, M.E.; Ghuman, S. Knowledge, practices, and attitudes of emergency contraception among female university students in KwaZulu-Natal, South Africa. *PLoS ONE* **2012**, *7*, e46346. [CrossRef]
24. Black, K.I.; Geary, R.; French, R.; Leefe, N.; Mercer, C.H.; Glasier, A.; Macdowall, W.; Gibson, L.; Datta, J.; Palmer, M.; et al. Trends in the use of emergency contraception in Britain: Evidence from the second and third National Surveys of Sexual Attitudes and Lifestyles. *BJOG* **2016**, *123*, 1600–1607. [CrossRef] [PubMed]
25. Chandna, A.; Nath, J.; Dhingra, D. Awareness of emergency contraception among 1st year medical students. *Int. J. Contemp. Med. Res.* **2016**, *3*. [CrossRef]
26. Lehan Mackin, M.; Clark, M.K.; McCarthy, A.M.; Farris, K. Knowledge and use of emergency contraception in college women. *West. J. Nurs. Res.* **2015**, *37*, 462–480. [CrossRef]
27. Shiferaw, B.Z.; Gashaw, B.T.; Tesso, F.Y. Factors associated with utilization of emergency contraception among female students in Mizan-Tepi University, South West Ethiopia. *BMC Res. Notes* **2015**, *8*, 817. [CrossRef]
28. Miller, L.M. College student knowledge and attitudes toward emergency contraception. *Contraception* **2011**, *83*, 68–73. [CrossRef] [PubMed]
29. Kgosiemang, B.; Blitz, J. Emergency contraceptive knowledge, attitudes and practices among female students at the University of Botswana: A descriptive survey. *Afr. J. Prim. Health Care Fam. Med.* **2018**, *10*, e1–e6. [CrossRef]
30. Bastianelli, C.; Rosato, E.; Farris, M.; Benagiano, G. Emergency contraception: A survey of 1773 women. *Eur. J. Contracept. Reprod. Health Care* **2016**, *21*, 455–461. [CrossRef] [PubMed]
31. Fontes, E.; Guerreiro, J.; Costa, T.; Miranda, A. Pattern of use of emergency oral contraception among Portuguese women. *Pharm. World Sci.* **2010**, *32*, 496–502. [CrossRef] [PubMed]
32. Collins, J.C.; Schneider, C.R.; Moles, R.J. Emergency contraception supply in Australian pharmacies after the introduction of ulipristal acetate: A mystery shopping mixed-methods study. *Contraception* **2018**, *98*, 243–246. [CrossRef] [PubMed]
33. Glasier, A.F.; Cameron, S.T.; Fine, P.M.; Logan, S.J.; Casale, W.; Van Horn, J.; Sogor, L.; Blithe, D.L.; Scherrer, B.; Mathe, H.; et al. Ulipristal acetate versus levonorgestrel for emergency contraception: A randomised non-inferiority trial and meta-analysis. *Lancet* **2010**, *375*, 555–562. [CrossRef]

34. Cwiak, C.; Howard, B.; Hsieh, J.; Ricciotti, N.; Sucato, G.S. Sexual and Contraceptive Behaviors among Adolescents Requesting Emergency Contraception. *J. Pediatr. Adolesc. Gynecol.* **2016**, *29*, 643–647. [CrossRef]
35. Bastianelli, C.; Farris, M.; Benagiano, G. Reasons for requesting emergency contraception: A survey of 506 Italian women. *Eur. J. Contracept. Reprod. Health Care* **2005**, *10*, 157–163. [CrossRef]
36. Chofakian, C.B.D.N.; Moreau, C.; Borges, A.L.V.; Santos, O.A.D. Contraceptive patterns after use of emergency contraception among female undergraduate students in Brazil. *Eur. J. Contracept. Reprod. Health Care* **2018**, *23*, 335–343. [CrossRef] [PubMed]
37. Hansen, C.C.; Svare, E.I.; Petersen, R.H.; Bock, J.E. Hvem anvender nødpraevention? [Who are the users of emergency contraception?]. *Ugeskr Laeger* **2002**, *164*, 5003–5005.
38. Frost, J.J.; Lindberg, L.D.; Finer, L.B. Young adults' contraceptive knowledge, norms and attitudes: Associations with risk of unintended pregnancy. *Perspect. Sex. Reprod. Health* **2012**, *44*, 107–116. [CrossRef] [PubMed]
39. Von Rosen, F.T.; von Rosen, A.J.; Müller-Riemenschneider, F.; Tinnemann, P. Awareness and knowledge regarding emergency contraception in Berlin adolescents. *Eur. J. Contracept. Reprod. Health Care* **2017**, *22*, 45–52. [CrossRef]
40. Veloso, D.L.; Peres, V.C.; Lopes, J.S.; Salge, A.K.; Guimarães, J.V. Anticoncepção de emergência: Conhecimento e atitude de acadêmicos de enfermagem [Emergency contraception: Knowledge and attitudes of nursing students]. *Rev. Gaucha Enferm* **2014**, *35*, 33–39. (In Portuguese) [CrossRef]
41. Cleland, K.; Raymond, E.G.; Westley, E.; Trussell, J. Emergency contraception review: Evidence-based recommendations for clinicians. *Clin. Obstet. Gynecol.* **2014**, *57*, 741–750. [CrossRef]
42. Raymond, E.G.; Halpern, V.; Lopez, L.M. Pericoital oral contraception with levonorgestrel: A systematic review. *Obstet. Gynecol.* **2011**, *117*, 673–681. [CrossRef] [PubMed]
43. Downing, A. University students' knowledge and attitudes toward emergency contraception pills. *J. Community Health Nurs.* **2014**, *31*, 75–89. [CrossRef]
44. Garrett, K.P.; Widman, L.; Francis, D.B.; Noar, S.M. Emergency contraception: Sources of information and perceptions of access among young adults. *Women Health* **2016**, *56*, 668–679. [CrossRef]
45. Davis, P.; Sarasveni, M.; Krishnan, J.; Bhat, L.D.; Kodali, N.K. Knowledge and attitudes about the use of emergency contraception among college students in Tamil Nadu, India. *J. Egypt. Public Health Assoc.* **2020**, *95*, 1. [CrossRef]
46. Richards, M.J.; Peters, M.; Sheeder, J.; Kaul, P. Contraception and Adolescent Males: An Opportunity for Providers. *J. Adolesc. Health* **2016**, *58*, 366–368. [CrossRef] [PubMed]
47. Coronado, P.J.; Delgado-Miguel, C.; Rey-Cañas, A.; Herráiz, M.A. Sexual and reproductive health in Spanish University Students. A comparison between medical and law students. *Sex. Reprod. Healthc.* **2017**, *11*, 97–101. [CrossRef] [PubMed]

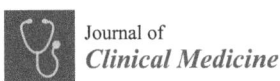

Article

Women's Access to Sexual and Reproductive Health Services during Confinement Due to the COVID-19 Pandemic in Spain

Fatima Leon-Larios [1], Isabel Silva Reus [2], Isabel Lahoz Pascual [3,*], José Cruz Quílez Conde [4], María José Puente Martínez [5], José Gutiérrez Ales [6] and Marta Correa Rancel [7,8]

1. Nursing Department, University of Seville, 41004 Seville, Spain; fatimaleon@us.es
2. Centro de Salud Sexual y Reproductiva de Villena, 03400 Alicante, Spain; isasilreus@gmail.com
3. Hospital Clínico Universitario Zaragoza, 50009 Zaragoza, Spain
4. Hospital Universitario de Basurto, 48013 Bilbao, Spain; jotxe_c@hotmail.com
5. Hospital San Pedro, 26006 Logroño, Spain; mjpuente@riojasalud.es
6. Hospital Universitario Virgen Macarena, 41009 Seville, Spain; jgales050655@gmail.com
7. Hospital Universitario de Canarias, 38320 Santa Cruz de Tenerife, Spain; tenerife1833@gmail.com
8. Departamento de Obstetricia-Ginecología, Pediatría, Preventiva, Medicina Legal y Forense, Microbiología, Parasitología, Universidad de la Laguna, 38200 Santa Cruz de Tenerife, Spain
* Correspondence: isalahoz@yahoo.com

Abstract: (1) Background: The COVID-19 pandemic has created a challenge for women's sexual and reproductive health care. The objective of this research was to analyse access to sexual and reproductive health services during confinement in Spain. (2) Methods: A descriptive and cross-sectional study was conducted with a random sample that was stratified by age in July and August 2020. (3) Results: A total of 1800 women were invited to participate, obtaining a response rate of 98.72%. The frequency of sexual relationships reduced during confinement. Counselling was offered both in person (30.7%) and telematically (39%), although there were also women who experienced access problems (30%). Of those women who required some LARC, only half had access to it, mainly due to the contact difficulties as a result of the limited number of consultations with their prescribing physicians. The use of emergency oral contraception and the use of services for the voluntary interruption of pregnancy were considerably reduced. The women who stated having been victims of gender-based violence were those that lived with their aggressors during confinement and had children. (4) Conclusions: It is necessary to ensure sexual and reproductive rights in confinement times and, for such a purpose, telemedicine can be a good tool that helps to avoid unmet contraceptive needs and unplanned pregnancies.

Keywords: contraception; COVID-19; LARC; emergency contraception; reproductive health; sexual health

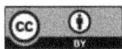

1. Introduction

On 14 March 2020, the state of alarm that imposed confinement of the population in Spain for 3 months was declared, limiting the provision of health services to those considered indispensable. According to a number of published studies, access to sexual and reproductive health services was affected in most countries worldwide [1,2]. The health-crisis situation that was created by COVID-19 produced an unprecedented scenario in health care, also exerting an impact on many women's sexual and reproductive health [3].

This new situation required scientific associations to adopt a stance on what would be considered unpostponable care provision. Consequently, in Spain, it was considered that the voluntary interruption of pregnancy, emergency contraception, suspected sexually transmitted infections, suspected severe complications associated with different contraceptive methods, and the care provided to victims of gender-based violence would be indispensable services. Undoubtedly, the challenge was related to counselling and the prescription of contraceptive methods via telephone calls or email messages [4–6], as well as access to contraceptive methods [3].

The report by the UN Population Fund had already warned that the measures used to fight against COVID-19 might leave 47 million of women without access to contraceptive methods worldwide [7,8]. In fact, the specific outcomes that are related to sexual and reproductive health in Spain reveal some of these challenges. The sale of contraceptive products recorded a strong reduction in the entire country.

The recommendation for the use Long-Acting Reversible Contraception (LARC) was that of choosing an alternative method and postponing the insertion of the IUD/implant. In relation to the withdrawal of these methods, the possibility of postponing extraction was considered due to the chance of extending it a little further based on need, and when their effectiveness could not be ensured, as well as concomitant use of a barrier method [8]. However, this policy was not adopted in all countries, as it was considered to be an essential service in some [7,9–12].

Predictions indicated that it might be a time in which a baby boom occurred, due to the limitation that some women might face in accessing contraceptive methods; however, according to the Spanish National Statistics Institute [13], no such increase took place, and the birth rate was reduced in the country [14].

On the other hand, the restrictions regarding displacement that were derived from the legislation that was in force at the time compelled women to spend the entire day at home, with many of them subject to potentially hazardous situations that may have been amplified due to the economic hardships faced by those who lost or had to adjust their jobs [3,15,16].

This research aims to analyse the events that took place regarding access to contraception methods and sexual and reproductive health services during the confinement that was caused by the SARS-CoV-19 pandemic in Spain.

2. Materials and Methods

A descriptive and cross-sectional study was conducted by means of a hetero-administered telephone survey managed by the SigmaDos survey company (Madrid, Spain). SigmaDos is an international Marketing and Public Survey Study company headquartered in Spain. Participants were contacted on their mobile and landline numbers. The participants were women aged between 15 and 49 years old and living in Spain. Those women who could not communicate in fluent Spanish were not included. Random sampling was performed by age quotas to ensure representativeness of the sample by age and region. The sample size was 1801 participants, with a possible error of +2.35% for a 95.5% confidence level (Sigma Two) and p/q = 50/50.

The data were collected in July and August 2020. The questionnaire included questions that were related to sociodemographic variables, namely: age, schooling level, relationship situation, income level, religious beliefs and nationality. In addition, the participants were asked questions that were related to their sexual habits and access to sexual and reproductive health services during confinement. The questionnaire was prepared by health professionals who specialized in sexual and reproductive health linked to Sociedad Española de Contracepción.

2.1. Statistical Analysis

For the categorical variables, the contingency tables were presented according to frequency and percentage values. Contingency tables with X^2 tests were prepared to examine the associations between categorical variables, and ϕ was reported to describe the effect size in each interrelation. A comparison of the means was performed by using the Student's test. SPSS for Mac (IBM Corp., Armonk, NY, USA), version 23.0, was used for the statistical analysis, considering *p*-values below 0.05 as significant.

2.2. Ethical Aspects

The women were free to stop answering questions at any moment. The Spanish health authorities do not require approval by a Research Ethics Committee for this type of study, in which the participants are asked to provide data about their sexual and contraceptive practices outside a health environment that establishes a professional relation. Confidentiality and anonymity were observed in the data treatment, and this is why IRB approval was not required. This study was conducted in accordance with the Declaration of Helsinki.

3. Results

A total of 1801 women took part in the study, with a final response rate of 98.72%, which represented 1778 women. The participants' sociodemographic characteristics are presented in Table 1. These characteristics are similar to the female general population in Spain. Most women lived with their partner, possessed a medium level of education, Spanish nationality and an average-low income level.

Table 1. Sociodemographic characteristics.

Variables	Total n (%) 1778 (100)
Age	
15–19 years old	170 (9.6)
20–24 years old	189 (10.6)
25–29 years old	211 (11.9)
30–34 years old	249 (14)
35–39 years old	308 (17.3)
40–44 years old	335 (18.8)
45–49 years old	316 (17.8)
Relationship situation	
Lives with her partner	1011 (56.9)
Steady partner, but not living together	325 (18.3)
No steady partner	442 (24.9)
Schooling level	
Elementary school	84 (4.7)
High school	917 (51.9)
University studies	767 (43.4)
Nationality	
Spanish	1602 (90.2)
Other	174 (9.8)
Income level	
Low	401 (25.8)
Average-low	663 (42.6)
Average	300 (19.3)
High	191 (12.3)

3.1. Sexual Habits

A total of 45% of the participants stated that the frequency of their sexual relationships was affected by the confinement during the pandemic. A total of 23.6% had not engaged in sexual relationships and 21.4% had reduced their frequency. However, 42% of the women were not affected by the new situation in terms of the frequency of their sexual relationships. The usual frequency in terms of sexual relationships was mostly maintained during confinement among the women who were aged at least 35 years old and in those that lived with their partners. It was precisely in these latter women where the highest increase was recorded (15.2%). A reduction was observed among the women who were aged less than 35 years old [$X^2(24) = 136.33$, $p < 0.001$, $\varphi = 0.283$], and in those that did not live with their steady partners [$X^2(8) = 730.31$, $p < 0.001$, $\varphi = 0.656$], as presented in Table 2.

Table 2. Frequency of sexual relationships during confinement in relation to age and relationship situation.

Sexual Relationships	Total n (%)	Age							Relationship Situation		
		15–19 n (%)	20–24 n (%)	25–29 n (%)	30–34 n (%)	35–39 n (%)	40–44 n (%)	45–49 n (%)	Lives with Her Partner n (%)	With a Partner, but Not Living Together n (%)	No Steady Partner n (%)
Increased	193 (11.3)	10 (8.5)	19 (10.4)	28 (13.4)	31 (12.6)	44 (14.5)	35 (10.6)	35 (8.3)	152 (15.2)	30 (9.6)	11 (2.8)
Reduced	362 (21.4)	31 (25.6)	56 (30.7)	49 (23.5)	57 (23.3)	51 (17.1)	65 (19.8)	65 (17.2)	175 (17.6)	102 (32.6)	85 (21.9)
Unchanged	169 (42.8)	15 (12.3)	51 (27.9)	88 (42.2)	104 (42.6)	143 (47.8)	157 (47.7)	157 (53.6)	620 (62.0)	63 (20.2)	44 (11.3)
No sexual relationships	400 (23.6)	64 (53.6)	55 (30.1)	44 (21.1)	52 (21.3)	60 (19.9)	66 (20.1)	66 (18.9)	38 (3.8)	117 (37.6)	244 (63.2)
DNK/DNA	17 (1.0)	0 (0.0)	2 (0.9)	0 (0.0)	1 (0.2)	2 (0.6)	6 (1.8)	6 (2.0)	13 (1.3)	0 (0.0)	3 (0.8)

3.2. Access to Contraceptive Methods

A total of 94% of the women had no need to resort to counselling or consultations about contraceptive methods during the confinement period, whereas 5% of the interviewees stated that they needed to access contraceptive counselling, as can be seen in Figure 1; of these, 30% failed to receive it, 39% were not able to access the service via telephone calls, and 30.7% did so in-person.

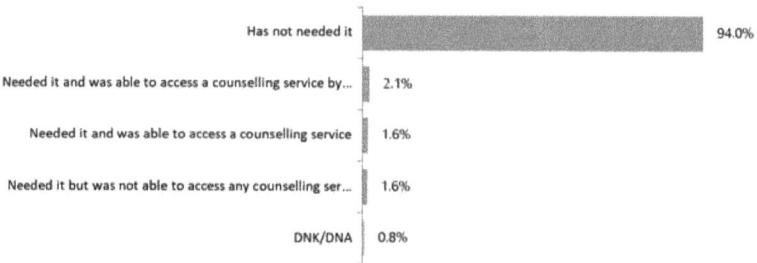

Figure 1. Access to counselling or consultations about contraceptive methods.

A total of 93.8% stated not having had any difficulty using or obtaining their usual contraceptive method during confinement. However, 4.4% of the women did experience such inconvenience. The most frequent reason why they faced difficulties to access their usual contraceptive method during confinement was not being able to renew the prescription due to the impossibility of contacting their prescribing physicians (63.3%), followed by dispensation problems in the pharmacies (18.3%). In addition, it was observed that those women who had more problems obtaining their usual method belonged to the age groups from 25 to 29 years old and from 30 to 34 years old: X^2 (12) = 30.51, p = 0.002, φ = 0.134.

A total of 95.1% of the women did not need to access any long-acting contraceptive method (IUD, implant) during confinement. Approximately half (48.15%) of the 3% that required a LARC method during this period were not able to access it.

A total of 2.8% of the women had to access and use the morning-after pill. This demand exceeded 5% among the women belonging to the age groups from 25 to 29 years old and from 35 to 39 years old: X^2(12) = 25.79, p = 0.011, φ = 0.123, as can be seen in Table 3. However, this is a considerably lower percentage than the habitual use rate in Spanish women, which is generally around 30–40%.

Table 3. Use of the emergency contraception pill (ECP) during confinement.

Have You Needed ECP?	Total n (%)	Age						
		15–19 n (%)	20–24 n (%)	25–29 n (%)	30–34 n (%)	35–39 n (%)	40–44 n (%)	45–49 n (%)
Yes	47 (2.8)	1 (1.1)	5 (3.0)	11 (5.5)	1 (0.3)	17 (5.6)	6 (1.9)	6 (1.8)
No	1646 (96.9)	118 (98.9)	177 (97.0)	197 (94.5)	243 (99.5)	282 (94.0)	323 (97.8)	306 (97.5)
DNK/DNA	0 (0.3)	0 (0.0)	0 (0.0)	0 (0.0)	1 (0.2)	1 (0.4)	1 (0.3)	5 (0.7)

3.3. Voluntary Interruption of Pregnancy

During 2020, the voluntary interruption of pregnancy (VIP) also recorded a decrease (17%), which represented a marked reduction during the confinement months. It was necessary to conduct the counselling sessions telematically and, frequently, to attend the clinic only once. Only Catalonia and Galicia implemented this by discontinuing the in-person counselling visits during confinement. It is not possible to establish if this decrease is related to access to services of VIP, or to the fact that less women needed the service.

3.4. Gender-Based Violence

During confinement, 2.2% of the women stated having experienced some situation of gender-based violence, especially those with lower schooling levels (7.2%) [$X^2(4) = 12.44$, $p = 0.014$, $\varphi = 0.086$]; lower income levels (4.7%) [$X^2(3) = 16.59$, $p = 0.001$, $\varphi = 0.105$]; with children (12.4%) [$X^2(6) = 12.63$, $p = 0.049$, $\varphi = 0.086$]; and those who were practicing Catholics (8%) [$X^2(6) = 44.79$, $p < 0.001$, $\varphi = 0.162$], as presented in Table 4. However, no differences were observed among the women who lived with their partners [$X^2(4) = 4.32$, $p = 0.364$]; by different age groups [$X^2(12) = 17.54$, $p = 0.130$]; or by nationality [$X^2(2) = 0.27$, $p = 0.874$], being not statistically significant.

Table 4. Factors associated with having being victims of gender-based violence during confinement.

Variables	Have You Been a Victim of Gender-Based Violence?	
	Yes n (%) 38 (2.2)	No n (%) 1649 (97.8)
Schooling level		
Elementary school	6 (7.6)	73 (92.4)
High school	19 (2.2)	836 (97.8)
University studies	13 (1.9)	740 (98.1)
Income level		
Low	18 (4.7)	366 (95.3)
Average-low	17 (2.5)	635 (97.5)
Average	2 (0.7)	290 (99.3)
High	0 (0)	185 (100)
Religious beliefs		
Practicing Catholic	19 (8)	214 (92)
Lapsed Catholic	8 (1.1)	708 (98.9)
Other religions	2 (1.6)	100 (98.4)
Agnostic/Atheist	9 (1.4)	635 (98.6)
Children		
Yes	21 (2.44)	839 (97.5)
No	17 (2)	817 (98)

4. Discussion

This research aimed at knowing women's experiences in Spain during the COVID-19 pandemic, regarding access to sexual and reproductive health services during the decreed confinement period. Questions were asked about access and counselling regarding usual contraception and emergency contraception, as well as whether they had experienced situations of gender-based violence.

Confinement ushered in some changes in women's lifestyles, with their sexual habits among them. As is the case in other studies, our results indicated that the frequency of sexual relationships was reduced among women [17,18], being even lower in those that did not live with their partners.

In our study, 5% of the participating women required contraceptive counselling during the pandemic, and of them, 3 out of 10 were not able to access it due to difficulties contacting their usual physicians, as already pointed out in the studies by Manze et al. [2] in the

USA and by Dema et al. [18] in the UK. These data are relatively higher than the data that were identified in Sweden, where few women had difficulties accessing contraceptive prescriptions and/or counselling [19]. However, these results must be interpreted considering that full confinement of the population was not implemented in Sweden, as was the case in Spain. Nevertheless, a reduction in the prescription of LARC methods was in fact identified in the aforementioned study, a result that is in line with what happened in Spain, with the possibility of having occurred in a higher number of unplanned pregnancies [19–21]. This might be because, unlike the case in other countries, it was not defined as an essential service in Spain [7].

Age was identified among the factors that were described in other studies, as well as people who reported risk behaviours as a risk factor for facing difficulties accessing the services [18,22].

In our research, the women who reported more difficulties accessing contraceptive methods were those belonging to the age group from 25 to 34 years old, coinciding with users of hormonal or LARC contraceptive methods. Our results indicated that 6 out of 10 women were able to access counselling on contraception with a health professional, whether in-person or via telephone calls. Use of the new technologies that comprise Telehealth is an alternative that would have to be considered as an option to meet the sexual and reproductive health needs of this collective, and such use should be increased in situations like those that were experienced during confinement, as already pointed out in previous studies [23–25]. Studies that have appraised the use of these alternatives to in-person visits have attested to their usefulness to ensure access to the services [18,21]. However, the results arising from this research indicate that some women were not able to have their demand met, as was the case in many countries [21]. However, the digital gap which might be experienced by the most vulnerable collective groups that were not educated on new technologies or lacked good quality access to the Internet should indeed be considered [26].

The use of emergency contraception during the pandemic was considerably reduced to unusual consumption values in Spain, where 3 out of 10 women resorted to emergency oral contraception [27]. Dispensation of emergency oral contraception products is free in pharmacies; therefore, their use and access by women should not have been compromised in Spain. However, these data are in line with what happened in other European countries where consumption was also reduced [28].

In a study that was conducted in 29 countries, access to abortion was limited in most of them during the COVID-19 pandemic [19].

The voluntary interruption of pregnancy was considered as an essential service during the pandemic, and bureaucracy was reduced to ease its provision to the women who required it in many countries [29]. However, the statistics showed a reduction in the number of abortions in Spain, a situation that was similar to that in other European countries [1,30], although an increase in the number of unsafe abortions was also verified [21]. Some European countries set out the proposal to increase pharmacological abortions to facilitate such provision to the women who needed them [31].

As predicted in some studies and reports, expressions of gender-based violence during the pandemic and confinement increased, despite the national statistics from many countries not reflecting such a rise [3,15,16]. The number of victims of gender-based violence was reduced by up to 8.4% during 2020 in Spain; the rate was 1.4 for every 1000 women aged at least 14 years old [32]. The highest reduction was recorded during the first two months of confinement, a trend that was maintained in the second part of 2020 in Spain [32]; however, it is unclear whether this decrease was real or was in fact driven by under-reporting due to the harsher confinement situation that was experienced by the victims with their aggressors. In the sample that comprises our research, 2 out of 100 women stated having experienced some situation of gender-based violence during confinement, with this being more frequent in those who lived with their partners and had children. At the global level, the reality indicated that the number of cases of gender-based violence increased with the COVID-19 pandemic [1].

Some of the strengths of this study lie in the sample size and its representativeness, as participation was high. This research allows identification of the weaknesses that were detected, in order to face them should confinement be implemented again. Among the limitations, we identified that it was not possible to establish a baseline that allowed us to compare the pre-pandemic situation with the experiences during confinement and, thus, establish comparisons. On the other hand, we assessed the access to sexual and reproductive health services, asking women about their perception of the situation experienced during the pandemic, though not based on access statistics.

5. Conclusions

The pandemic exerted a negative impact on women's sexual and reproductive health, exposing them to risk situations for unplanned pregnancies by not having access to the usual services that were provided prior to the pandemic, and that were now limited. Access to LARCs was considerably reduced and delayed. It is necessary to integrate the difficulties that were identified by the women in accessing sexual and reproductive health services, as well as to ensure sexual and reproductive rights through the provision of these services. For such a purpose, the suggestion is to enhance and strengthen Telemedicine with resources that enable an efficient response in situations of confinement or restrictions, regarding access to health services in similar situations in the future.

Author Contributions: Conceptualization, methodology and software, M.C.R., J.G.A., J.C.Q.C. and M.J.P.M.; formal analysis, F.L.-L., I.S.R. and I.L.P.; writing—original draft preparation, F.L.-L., M.C.R. and I.L.P. All authors have read and agreed to the published version of the manuscript.

Funding: This research received no external funding. This research was funded by Sociedad Española de Contracepción. The APC was also funded by Sociedad Española de Contracepción.

Institutional Review Board Statement: The study was conducted in accordance with the Declaration of Helsinki. Ethical review and approval were waived for this study since the subjects were invited to participate voluntarily.

Informed Consent Statement: Informed consent was obtained from all the subjects that were involved in the study. Written informed consent was obtained from the participants to publish this paper.

Data Availability Statement: The datasets that support the findings of this study are available from the corresponding author upon reasonable written request.

Acknowledgments: We would like to thank the former board of Sociedad Española de Contracepción for their contribution to this research, especially Paloma Lobo Abascal, Jose Ramón Serrano Navarro and José Vicente González Navarro, who participated in the design of the questionnaire. We also wish to thank Sociedad Española de Contracepción for their support in publishing this paper.

Conflicts of Interest: The authors declare no conflict of interest.

References

1. Endler, M.; Al-Haidari, T.; Benedetto, C.; Chowdhury, S.; Christilaw, J.; El Kak, F.; Galimberti, D.; Garcia-Moreno, C.; Gutierrez, M.; Ibrahim, S.; et al. How the coronavirus disease 2019 pandemic is impacting sexual and reproductive health and rights and response: Results from a global survey of providers, researchers, and policy-makers. *Acta Obstet. Gynecol. Scand.* **2021**, *100*, 571–578. [CrossRef] [PubMed]
2. Manze, M.; Romero, D.; Johnson, G.; Pickering, S. Factors related to delays in obtaining contraception among pregnancy-capable adults in New York state during the COVID-19 pandemic: The CAP study. *Sex. Reprod. Healthc.* **2022**, *31*, 100697. [CrossRef]
3. Kumar, N. COVID-19 era: A beginning of upsurge in unwanted pregnancies, unmet need for contraception and other women related issues. *Eur. J. Contracept. Reprod. Health Care* **2020**, *25*, 323–325. [CrossRef] [PubMed]
4. Nanda, K.; Lebetkin, E.; Steiner, M.J.; Yacobson, I.; Dorflinger, L.J. Contraception in the Era of COVID-19. *Glob. Health Sci. Pract.* **2020**, *8*, 166–168. [CrossRef] [PubMed]
5. Hurtado, A.C.M.; Crowley, S.M.; Landry, K.M.; Landry, M.S. Telehealth Contraceptive Care in 2018: A Quality Improvement Study of Barriers to Access and Patient Satisfaction. *Contraception* **2022**, in press. [CrossRef] [PubMed]

6. Riley, T.; Sully, E.; Ahmed, Z.; Biddlecom, A. Estimates of the potential impact of the COVID-19 pandemic on sexual and reproductive health in low- and middle-income countries. *Int. Perspect. Sex. Reprod. Health* **2020**, *46*, 73–76. [CrossRef]
7. Bateson, D.J.; Lohr, P.A.; Norman, W.V.; Moreau, C.; Gemzell-Danielsson, K.; Blumenthal, P.D.; Hoggart, L.; Li, H.-W.R.; Aiken, A.R.; Black, K.I. The impact of COVID-19 on contraception and abortion care policy and practice: Experiences from selected countries. *BMJ Sex. Reprod. Health* **2020**, *46*, 241–243. [CrossRef]
8. Weinberger, M.; Hayes, B.; White, J.; Skibiak, J. Doing Things Differently: What It Would Take to Ensure Continued Access to Contraception During COVID-19. *Glob. Health Sci. Pract.* **2020**, *8*, 169–175. [CrossRef]
9. Society of Obstetricians and Gynecologists of Canada (SOGC). COVID-19 Resources. 2020. Available online: https://sogc.org/en/content/COVID-19/COVID-19.aspx?COVIDResources=2 (accessed on 25 April 2022).
10. Royal College of Obstetricians and Gynaecologists. *Coronavirus (COVID-19) Infection and Abortion Care*; Royal College of Obstetricians and Gynaecologists: London, UK, 2020.
11. Royal Australian and New Zealand College of Obstetricians and Gynaecologists (RANZCOG). Coronavirus (COVID-19): Information Hub. 2020. Available online: https://ranzcog.edu.au/news/covid-19-anti-d-and-abortion (accessed on 1 May 2022).
12. Faculty of Sexual & Reproductive Healthcare (FSRH). Essential Services in Sexual and Reproductive Healthcare. 2020. Available online: https://www.fsrh.org/fsrh-and-covid-19-resourcesand-information-for-srh/ (accessed on 28 April 2022).
13. Instituto Nacional de Estadística. Tasa de Embarazos. 2020. Available online: https://www.ine.es/jaxiT3/Datos.htm?t=1433 (accessed on 28 April 2022).
14. Aassve, A.; Cavalli, N.; Mencarini, L.; Plach, S.; Sanders, S. Early assessment of the relationship between the COVID-19 pandemic and births in high-income countries. *Proc. Natl. Acad. Sci. USA* **2021**, *118*, e2105709118. [CrossRef]
15. United Nations. Policy Brief: The Impact of COVID-19 on Women. Available online: https://unsdg.un.org/resources/policy-brief-impact-covid-19-women (accessed on 28 April 2022).
16. Impact of the COVID-19 Pandemic on Family Planning and Ending Gender-Based Violence, Female Genital Mutilation and Child Marriage. UNFPA Interim Technical Note. Available online: https://www.unfpa.org/sites/default/files/resource-pdf/COVID-19_impact_brief_for_UNFPA_24_April_2020_1.pdf (accessed on 28 April 2022).
17. Lete, I.; Novalbos, J.; de la Viuda, E.; Lugo, F.; Herrero, M.; Obiol, M.; Perelló, J.; Sanchez-Borrego, R. Impact of the Lockdown Due to COVID-19 Pandemic in the Use of Combined Hormonal Oral Contraception in Spain—Results of a National Survey: Encovid. *Open Access J. Contracept.* **2021**, *12*, 103–111. [CrossRef]
18. Dema, E.; Gibbs, J.; Clifton, S.; Copas, A.J.; Tanton, C.; Riddell, J.; Pérez, R.B.; Reid, D.; Bonell, C.; Unemo, M.; et al. Initial impacts of the COVID-19 pandemic on sexual and reproductive health service use and unmet need in Britain: Findings from a quasi-representative survey (Natsal-COVID). *Lancet Public Health* **2022**, *7*, e36–e47. [CrossRef]
19. Hultstrand, J.N.; Törnroos, E.; Gemzell-Danielsson, K.; Larsson, M.I.; Makenzius, M.; Sundström-Poromaa, I.; Tydén, T.; Ragnar, M.E. Induced abortion and access to contraception in Sweden during the COVID-19 pandemic. *BMJ Sex. Reprod. Health* **2022**. *ahead of print*. [CrossRef] [PubMed]
20. Walker, S.H. Effect of the COVID-19 pandemic on contraceptive prescribing in general practice: A retrospective analysis of English prescribing data between 2019 and 2020. *Contracept. Reprod. Med.* **2022**, *7*, 3. [CrossRef]
21. Aly, J.; Haeger, K.O.; Christy, A.Y.; Johnson, A.M. Contraception access during the COVID-19 pandemic. *Contracept. Reprod. Med.* **2020**, *5*, 17. [CrossRef] [PubMed]
22. Diamond-Smith, N.; Logan, R.; Marshall, C.; Corbetta-Rastelli, C.; Gutierrez, S.; Adler, A.; Kerns, J. COVID-19's impact on contraception experiences: Exacerbation of structural inequities in women's health. *Contraception* **2021**, *104*, 600–605. [CrossRef]
23. Sturgiss, E.; Dut, G.M.; Matenge, S.; Desborough, J.; Dykgraaf, S.H.; Mazza, D.; Kidd, M. COVID-19 and access to sexual and reproductive healthcare for young people: An overview of the international literature and policy. *Aust. J. Gen. Pract.* **2022**, *51*, 271–277. [CrossRef] [PubMed]
24. Lindberg, L.D.; Bell, D.L.; Kantor, L.M. The Sexual and Reproductive Health of Adolescents and Young Adults During the COVID-19 Pandemic. *Perspect. Sex. Reprod. Health* **2020**, *52*, 75–79. [CrossRef] [PubMed]
25. Bryson, A.; Koyama, A.; Hassan, A. Addressing long-acting reversible contraception access, bias, and coercion: Supporting adolescent and young adult reproductive autonomy. *Curr. Opin. Pediatr.* **2021**, *33*, 345–353. [CrossRef]
26. Shaikh, I.; Küng, S.A.; Aziz, H.; Sabir, S.; Shabbir, G.; Ahmed, M.; Dabash, R. Telehealth for Addressing Sexual and Reproductive Health and Rights Needs During the COVID-19 Pandemic and Beyond: A Hybrid Telemedicine-Community Accompaniment Model for Abortion and Contraception Services in Pakistan. *Front. Glob. Womens Health* **2021**, *2*, 705262. [CrossRef]
27. Leon-Larios, F.; Ruiz-Ferron, C.; Jalon-Neira, R.M.; Praena-Fernández, J.M. Nursing Students' Knowledge, Awareness, and Experiences of Emergency Contraception Pills' Use. *J. Clin. Med.* **2022**, *11*, 418. [CrossRef]
28. Roland, N.; Drouin, J.; Desplas, D.; Duranteau, L.; Cuenot, F.; Dray-Spira, R.; Weill, A.; Zureik, M. Impact of Coronavirus disease 2019 (COVID-19) on contraception use in 2020 and up until the end of April 2021 in France. *Contraception* **2022**, *108*, 50–55. [CrossRef] [PubMed]
29. Raymond, E.G.; Grossman, D.; Mark, A.; Upadhyay, U.D.; Dean, G.; Creinin, M.D.; Coplon, L.; Perritt, J.; Atrio, J.M.; Taylor, D.; et al. Commentary: No-test medication abortion: A sample protocol for increasing access during a pandemic and beyond. *Contraception* **2020**, *101*, 361–366. [CrossRef] [PubMed]
30. Registro Estatal de Interrupciones Voluntarias del Embarazo. Dirección General de Salud Pública. Available online: https://www.sanidad.gob.es/profesionales/saludPublica/prevPromocion/embarazo/tablas_figuras.htm#Figura1 (accessed on 28 April 2022).

31. Cioffi, A.; Cioffi, F.; Rinaldi, R. COVID-19 and abortion: The importance of guaranteeing a fundamental right. *Sex. Reprod. Healthc.* **2020**, *25*, 100538. [CrossRef] [PubMed]
32. Instituto Nacional de Estadística. Estadística de Violencia Doméstica y Violencia de Género. Available online: https://www.ine.es/prensa/evdvg_2020.pdf (accessed on 28 April 2022).

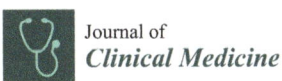

Review

How Does Contraceptive Use Affect Women's Sexuality? A Novel Look at Sexual Acceptability

Salvatore Caruso *, Gaia Palermo, Giuseppe Caruso and Agnese Maria Chiara Rapisarda

Research Group for Sexology, Department of General Surgery and Medical Surgical Specialties, Gynecological Clinic, University of Catania, Via Santa Sofia, 78, 95125 Catania, Italy; gaia.palermo.17@gmail.com (G.P.); giu.caruso97@gmail.com (G.C.); rapisardaagnesemc@gmail.com (A.M.C.R.)
* Correspondence: scaruso@unict.it

Abstract: Among the components of a healthy life, sexuality is essential, contributing to both the psychophysical and social well-being of women and, consequently, to their quality of life. A poorly investigated standpoint is the acceptability of contraceptive methods, both in terms of their tolerability and metabolic neutrality and in terms of their impact on sexual life. In this context, we will provide an overview of the different methods of contraception and their effects on female sexuality, from biological changes to organic, social, and psychological factors, which can all shape sexuality. A MEDLINE/PubMed review of the literature between 2010 and 2021 was conducted using the following key words and phrases: hormonal contraception, contraceptives, female sexual function, libido, sexual arousal and desire, and sexual pain. Recent studies have supported the effects of contraceptives on women's sexuality, describing a variety of positive and negative events in several domains of sexual function (desire, arousal, orgasm, pain, enjoyment). However, satisfaction with sexual activity depends on factors that extend beyond sexual functioning alone. A more holistic approach is needed to better understand the multitude of factors linked to women's sexuality and contraception. Contraceptive counseling must consider these important elements since they are closely related to good compliance and maximize non-contraceptive health benefits.

Keywords: hormonal contraception; long-acting reversible contraceptive; quality of life; sexual arousal and desire; sexual behavior; short-acting reversible contraceptive

1. Introduction

Reproductive and sexual health represent a human right that has to be defended and preserved. The aim of contraception is to avoid undesired pregnancies and assure a satisfying sexual life free from procreative risks.

The successful control of fertility steers a woman toward great benefits from personal, economic, and cultural autonomy to psychological and physical welfare [1].

A holistic approach to contraceptive requirements has to consider the individual's reproductive and sexual health needs. Physicians should use simple, understandable language when counseling about potential risks, benefits, and uncertainties to enable women to choose the best contraceptive for themselves. Counseling is mainly aimed at supporting women's choices. Different variables can affect the choice of contraceptive and include the woman's subjective characteristics, as well as the ready availability and straightforward usage of the method [2].

The main goal of modern contraception has been to allow the woman and her partner to live the sexual experience free from the worry of an unwanted pregnancy. Although these are good intentions, at least at the beginning of the use of hormonal contraception, possible interference with the quality of sexual life, desire, arousal, and the level of acceptability in women using hormonal contraceptives has not been well investigated. In the past, few investigations have reported whether hormonal contraception can positively or negatively affect the sexual function of users in different domains of female sexuality, such as desire, arousal, orgasm, lubrication, enjoyment, and pain [3].

However, it is important to emphasize that many factors beyond sexual function itself influence satisfaction with sexual activity. In fact, if sociocultural variables can modulate female sexuality in its qualitative and quantitative aspects, on the one hand, it is also true that the hormonal changes promoted by hormonal contraception could influence sexual habits [3]. Physiologically, in women who do not use hormonal contraceptives or who have taken non-hormonal contraceptives, sexual desire increases during the periovulatory phase of the menstrual cycle [4]. At midcycle, the gradual increase in estrogen promotes the thinning of the cervical mucus, which results in watery secretion with low viscoelasticity. Moreover, androgens are required for the synthesis of the glycoproteins needed for mucous formation [5]; this may explain the decreased vaginal lubrication noted by some women when they are using a hormonal contraceptive with antiandrogenic activity. In addition, hypoandrogenism may cause the onset of vulvodynia and contribute to impaired vaginal lubrication [6,7]. On the other hand, the increase in progesterone during the luteal phase promotes mucus reduction, with less water and a barrier to sperm cells [8]. The increase in cervical mucus and vaginal lubrication may activate the phase of genital arousal, which could b capable of centrally turning on sexual interest [9].

Over the past decade, an increasing number of studies have been engaged in investigating the influences of contraception on sexuality and, above all, the association between hormonal contraception and libido [10].

Even so, a global approach is necessary to study the many facets of female sexuality and the influence of contraception on users. Investigating these issues with greater interest than what has been shown up to now could bring benefits to female sexual well-being and foster a wider use of hormonal contraception.

In this review, we will focus on the different methods of contraception based on their steroid compounds, the route of administration, and regimen, as well as their impact on female sexuality, extrapolated from the most recent literature articles.

2. Materials and Methods

We conducted a comprehensive search of the literature using MEDLINE and PubMed. The research covered the period from 2011 to 2021. We used combinations of the following search terms: female sexual function, hormonal contraception, libido, long-acting reversible contraceptive, quality of life and short-acting reversible contraceptive, sexual arousal and desire disorders, sexual pain, and sexual behavior. Titles and abstracts were reviewed by the authors to assess their relevance to the review. Eligibility criteria also included a comparison between two or more contraceptive methods and their influence on female sexual health and the change in users' quality of life. The following criteria were used to exclude articles: unpublished reports, unspecified date, and the site of the study or suspicion of duplicate reporting. Efforts were made to ensure that there was no overlap within the results and that no case was counted twice. Variables extracted and analyzed included an improvement or deterioration in sexual health—mainly of desire, arousal, lubrication, and sexual pain.

This systematic review had no "stand-alone" study protocol. For reporting outcomes for the ongoing study, the PRISMA guidelines were adopted [Appendix A, Figure A1].

3. Results

We analyzed more than one hundred abstracts; however, the quality of sexual life, desire, arousal, and the level of acceptability of hormonal contraception in women were not well investigated.

3.1. Combined Oral Contraception and Sexuality

Over the last fifty years, many studies have been drawn up on cultural and social aspects related to hormonal contraceptives [11].

Firstly, the impact of "the pill" on society has been misunderstood. Despite all the social and moral controversies and the scientific debate on side effects, hormonal contraception has, nowadays, obtained a consolidated role [12]. Combined oral contraception (COC) is a reasonable and reversible method of contraception, available with a wide modality of administration and a wide choice of doses of administration, formulations, and regimens.

COC could have advantages in female sexuality, including increasing intra-partner satisfaction and the number of instances of sexual intercourse; resolving painful gynecological symptoms, such as those due to dysmenorrhea or endometriosis, or bothersome symptoms, such as menorrhagia and alterations in the menstrual cycle; and improving the signs and symptoms of clinical hyperandrogenisms, such as acne and hirsutism [13]. However, it could have disadvantages in relation to sexual desire, arousal, lubrication, pain, and orgasm. In fact, sexual side effects are considered to be among the factors promoting contraceptive discontinuation or switching [14].

Hypoactive sexual desire disorder is the most frequently reported sexual symptom among women using hormonal contraception. In a study of 3740 women, the authors observed that 43% of them had experienced a reduction in sexual desire attributed to the use of hormonal contraceptives, compared with 12% of women who used hormone-free contraceptives [15].

To support these data, there is also an Egyptian study on 8422 women using progestin-only contraceptives, in which a significant general worsening in sexuality in terms of desire, arousal, lubrication, and orgasm was reported.

Smaller concentrations of estrogens and progestogen with antiandrogenic activity can lead to vulvo-vaginal atrophy due to reduced activation of sex steroid receptors in the case of a relative lack of estrogen; conversely, the effects of reduced androgen concentrations have not yet been elucidated [16]. On the other hand, current hormonal contraception is characterized by a frankly antiandrogenic pharmacological activity due to the characteristics of both estrogen and progestin [17].

According to recent studies, the dose of ethinylestradiol (EE) can affect the blood levels of free testosterone (FT), reducing it below a critical threshold on the basis of its dosage, and potentially leading to at least one group of women (those most sensitive to steroid variations) suffering from hypoactive sexual desire [18]. Its activity is coupled with the anti-androgenic activity of progestogen [19].

Just over 10 years ago, COCs containing natural estrogen, namely estradiol valerate (E2V) and 17β-estradiol (17β-E), were marketed. E2V and (17β-E) have a lower impact than EE on the synthesis of hepatic proteins, such as the sex hormone-binding globulin (SHBG) [20–22].

The assumption of a detrimental effect of the antiandrogenic progestogen on female sexual function was challenged by the STABLE study, a multicenter, randomized, double-blind study on either E2V/dienogest (DNG) or EE/levonorgestrel (LNG). Both treatments were associated with a significant increase in the sexual function of the users between baseline and end-of-study, and resulted in similar improvements in desire, arousal, satisfaction, orgasm, and lubrication [23]. The authors supported the non-difference in sexual function to be due to the progestin component, dienogest with antiandrogenic activity, and levonorgestrel with androgenic activity. They deduced that both formulations had the same effects on sexual function. They did not consider the effects of the two estrogens, E2V and EE, on the modulation of plasma SHBG levels. E2V has a lower estrogenic effect than EE. Therefore, it can be hypothesized that the increase in SHBG is more reduced in the contraceptives with E2V than in those with EE. Hence, hypoandrogenism appears less marked despite the antiandrogenic properties of DNG [20,22].

These results are consistent with other studies investigating the effect of E2V/DNG on the quality of sex life of women who requested a contraceptive to avoid pregnancy [24]. Finally, hypoandrogenism induced by E2V/DNG is milder than that of other COCs containing EE combined with progestogen with antiandrogenic activity [21]. This could be caused by two mechanisms as follows: EE can raise the level of the SHBG and consequent decrease in FT; however, it can directly suppress the ovary androgen production [25]. Moreover, continuous or extended regimens of administration have been associated with supplementary positive variation in a multitude of sexual acceptability factors, from sexual function and libido to a reduction in dysmenorrhea, duration of withdrawal bleeds, and breast tenderness [18]. It is also true that most of the users of hormonal contraceptives do not undergo a reduction in libido even though, in most studies, a decline in plasma levels of FT and an increase in SHBG were demonstrated [26]. Pastor et al., showed that libido decreased only in women using oral contraceptives that contained 15 µg of EE but not in those using COCs containing 20 or 35 µg of EE. Nonetheless, the reduction in vaginal lubrication with sexual arousal disorder reported by some users could be due to the low peripheral dose of EE [27]. Experiencing reduced desire seems to be a strong predictor for changing or suspending a contraceptive method [28].

On the other hand, several studies correlate the use of COCs with changes in sexual function—particularly sexual desire and arousal, frequency of sexual activity, and orgasm achievement—but not with enjoyment of sexual activity [28,29].

However, it is still unclear whether these changes in sexuality are directly related to hormonal effects or pill-induced mood swings, or are primarily psychological rejection reactions to fertility control [26].

Another factor that can positively influence women's sexuality is the certainty of not wanting children. Hormonal contraceptives are a highly effective form of contraception; they help to eliminate anxiety related to the fear of pregnancy, encouraging an easier and more enjoyable sexual experience. Differences in terms of anti-androgenic results and influence on sexuality could be attributed, in part, to the known effects of estrogen on SHBG synthesis and, in part, to the androgenic or anti-androgenic activity of the involved progestin [30]. In conclusion, every woman has her own sensitivity to sexual steroids; therefore, it is not possible to simplify the contraceptive choice. Thus, an effort is strongly required to adopt a hormonal contraceptive that is adapted to her subjective needs. It is essential that counseling considers the woman's expectations concerning the effects of hormonal contraception on her own sexual activity. In fact, most women expect an improvement in sexuality while they are on hormonal contraception; a worsening or lack of change could lead to discontinuation [31].

3.2. Vaginal Ring and Sexuality

The contraceptive vaginal ring (CVR) is an appropriate method for women with indications for hormonal contraception (HC) who have previously experienced sexual dysfunction using oral contraceptives [32].

Many studies that compare COCs and CVRs report that there is no difference in terms of efficacy to inhibit ovulation. The only difference is the compliance of women, maybe also thanks to the elimination of daily intake [33].

Some authors have shown that CVR, in addition to contraceptive efficacy, could promote a positive effect on the couple's sexuality as a whole, and amplify the complicity and satisfaction of both the partners [34].

Furthermore, in previous studies, women using CVR had better outcomes in relation to desire and sexual satisfaction compared with women using oral hormonal contraceptives. In fact, CVR users had higher sexual desire than those using oral contraceptives combined with EE or desogestrel-only pills [35].

In addition, other authors evaluated sexual efficacy and function by a prospective study involving a prolonged regimen of CVR. An improvement in sexual function and a reduction in sexual discomfort were observed after two months of use [36].

Unlike these, other investigations obtained conflicting results. Indeed, decreased sexual desire was observed more frequently in women using CVR than in those who were intaking oral contraceptives containing 30 µg of EE and 3 mg of DRSP [37]. Today, new polymer compositions are produced for use in the manufacture of CVRs. Their characteristic is to give greater stability and a better withdrawal of steroids from the CVR.

In addition to having reduced adverse events, such as spotting, the users report a better QoL and better sexual function when interviewed [38].

In favor of these data, there are many comparisons between the vaginal ring, other types of contraception, and no hormonal contraception. Some authors concluded, from the results, that women who use HC through any route of administration experience an improvement in their sexuality, evidenced by positive variations of sexual interest and fantasies and orgasm intensity and satisfaction; they supported such an improvement by relating it to the reduction in their anxiety and discomfort during unprotected sex of women before starting HC [23,39].

All studies cited relate to the once-a-month ring through which 15 mg of EE and 120 mg of etonogestrel are released daily.

3.3. Progestin-Only Pill (POP) and Sexuality

The most common contraceptive used in Europe during breastfeeding is a POP that contains low doses of desogestrel. Clinical trials of POPs have proved no effects on breastfeeding performance and, consequently, no harmful events in breastfed newborns [39]. Authors noted in a double-blind, placebo-controlled study that POP users have no adverse effects on sexual function compared to women using HC. Overall, data provide reassurance that POPs are unlikely to have a major impact on sexual desire [40]. However, some authors have postulated that progestogen POPs with antiandrogenic activity may adversely affect sexual interest and fantasies. The findings of the studies reinforce the hypothesis that that the effect on sexual function depends on the particular type of progestin and not its dosage [41]. Reports correlating a levonorgestrel-containing combined contraceptive with a desogestrel-containing one have shown different impacts on SHBG concentrations [42]. Moreover, it has been proposed that desogestrel, for its androgenic activity, may exert positive effects on libido [43]. The question of how a different dose or type of progestin could contrastingly affect female sexuality is worthy of additional research.

3.4. Intrauterine Devices and Sexuality

The high contraceptive efficacy of long-acting reversible contraceptives (LARC) is the most important characteristic of this kind of intrauterine device. For this reason, they are widely used in current programs and policies of family planning [44]. Nowadays, women who use SARCs, such as oral, patch, or vaginal combined hormonal contraceptives, or non-hormonal contraceptives, and who have had incorrect or discontinued use in their history, with the risk of having an unwanted pregnancy, could adopt an intrauterine device [45].

An important aspect that could influence and prolong happiness with an intrauterine device is sexual acceptability. Cramps, pain, and bleeding are the most commonly cited reasons from women for discontinuation within the first 12 months, even if they are adverse events that usually appear during the first months of use [46]. The partner could also influence the acceptability of the intrauterine device when he experiences bad sex due to the perception of the intrauterine device string during intercourse [47]. Conversely, the absence of systemic hormonal repercussions makes these intrauterine devices neutral on sexual libido compared to other hormonal methods [48]. However, authors have shown by their investigation that the QoL and sexual function improve after LNG-IUS placement. Moreover, the reduction in dysmenorrhea is another important reported aspect [44,49].

Both frequency of sexual activity and sexual enjoyment are positively related to satisfaction with a contraceptive method, as is demonstrated in other studies [50,51]. High standards of satisfaction [50] and a better QoL [52,53] have been described in IUD users who previously had unwanted pregnancies using a SARC. Furthermore, authors observed that women with sexual dysfunction experience significant improvement in sexual desire, arousal, orgasm, and overall sexual function while using LNG-IUS. Moreover, a cross-sectional investigation observed that sexual symptoms in women using LNG-IUS were the same [54] or higher than women who adopted a copper intrauterine device (IUD) [55].

These data are also supported by other recent studies in which healthy women who were using IUD for long-term contraception were enrolled. Among them, half used LNG-IUSs as the study group and the other half used copper IUDs. There was no significant difference in the individual score and the total scores of questionnaires used to investigate sexual function between the groups [50,56]. At first, intrauterine devices were not thought to be proper for adolescents until observational studies not only showed their contraceptive safety but also their positive role in sexuality. Therefore, new, smaller devices have encouraged doctors to suggest, and adolescents to use, intrauterine contraception. Finally, intrauterine devices do not appear to have negative interference during sexual experience, due to the absence of systemic steroid effects and the fact that they maintain the natural expression of sexuality and enjoyment during sexual intercourse [57].

3.5. Progestin Contraceptive Implant and Sexuality

Progestin-only contraceptive implants (POI) are subdermal devices composed of a total of 68 mg of etonogestrel (ENG), which is liberated daily at low doses of 25–70 µg on the subdermal tissue of the arm. It has the advantage of being discreet and easy to use and is classified as a LARC [58]. Some studies showed an improvement in QoL and no negative effects on libido and sexual function [54,59]. Relevant benefits to sexual function were also observed, consisting of increase in sexual pleasure, personal initiative, orgasm experience, and satisfaction; authors argued that these benefits were due to decreased anxiety and discomfort [60]. In comparative studies, greater sexual interest was observed in users of RNG implants than in users of oral contraceptives [61].

4. Conclusions

Today, the topic "sexuality and contraception" is a much debated field of study. It is not easy to correlate the sexual benefits or discomforts with hormonal contraception considering only the objective/biological side effects. Psychological influences can intervene before, during, and after the use of the contraceptive, hormonal or not, promoting benefits or producing no changes in sexual function [14].

During the counseling to prescribe a contraceptive, the health care practitioner (HCP) should investigate the woman's quality of sexual life, so as to work out the method that could maintain or improve her sexuality together. At the follow-up, shared with the user in a timely manner, it will be necessary to reassess the impact of the adopted method on sexuality, and, if disturbing effects on sexuality are highlighted, opt for another contraceptive. Again, the choice of a new method must take into account the woman's propensity and its impact on sexual function. Not infrequently, women may manifest anxiety when they experience their sexuality disturbed by the hormonal contraceptive. A review of a temporal association between the baseline of female sexual dysfunction and the introduction of contraception is warranted, as is an assessment of the bio-psycho-social exemplar of other implicit contributing elements. Attributing a sexual dysfunction to the use of a contraceptive is to be avoided at all costs. The contraceptive could also cause a sexological disorder. Researching the correct dysfunctional causes often involves an interdisciplinary approach. In fact, pain during vaginal intercourse, marital conflict, medical surgical comorbidities, or a history of sexual abuse may emerge during contraceptive counseling. A specialist consultation must be requested for each of them.

For all these reasons, developments in oral contraception are continuing. One hormonal contraceptive cannot be the solution to all problems. In our experience, COCs containing E2 are an innovation that avoids CHC discontinuation in women suffering from acquired hypoactive sexual desire disorder during CHC intake with hypoandrogenic effects [21].

Consequently, the concept that all women are different and variably sensitive to COC steroids has to be emphasized; in fact, we are going into a historical period in which the principal concept is to advise a COC tailored to particular women. Therefore, the first step in prescribing a COC is to understand the needs of the subject and to explore her current sexual health.

Beyond the changes in sexual function secondary to the effects of hormonal contraception, there are gray areas regarding the qualitative changes in sexual pleasure during contraceptive use. Some authors support the hypothesis that a woman's contraceptive choice plays a role in the contraceptive effects on sexual experience and pleasure [62]. There are women who experience discomfort in being aware that they are using a contraceptive method during sex or feeling the intravaginal ring during intercourse [63].

Others consider these perceptions to favor a positive effect on the sexuality of the couple as a whole [34].

These behaviors can be generalized to all contraceptive users, nominally LARCs and SARCs. In fact, users are able to customize the use of the method while maintaining its effectiveness and to adapt it to their sexuality [64].

Sexual function in reproductive-age women can depend on the influence of sex hormones as well as on psychological, sociocultural, and relationship influences. Studies on the sexual dysfunction in women using hormonal contraceptives are single-center studies, and there are no prospective studies. Large cross-sectional and longitudinal studies have not identified a correlation between hormonal contraceptives and sexual function in women. Steroids may have a modifying effect on sexual function, but social influences are just as important [65].

Even if healthcare professionals are adequately trained to treat endocrine and gynecological disorders with hormonal contraceptives, such as chronic pelvic pain, dysmenorrhea, or hyperandrogenism, there may be evident gaps in addressing their patients' sexual distress or sex disorder. To overcome these gaps, it is necessary to train healthcare professionals in sexual medicine and to promote better sexual well-being, including in the contraceptive field.

Author Contributions: Conceptualization, methodology and data curation, S.C.; investigation and writing—original draft preparation, G.P. and G.C.; writing—review editing and visualization, G.P. and A.M.C.R. All authors have read and agreed to the published version of the manuscript.

Funding: This research received no external funding.

Institutional Review Board Statement: Not applicable.

Informed Consent Statement: Not applicable.

Data Availability Statement: No new data were created or analyzed in this study. Data sharing is not applicable to this article.

Acknowledgments: We wish to thank the Scientific Bureau of the University of Catania for language support.

Conflicts of Interest: The authors declare no conflict of interest.

Appendix A

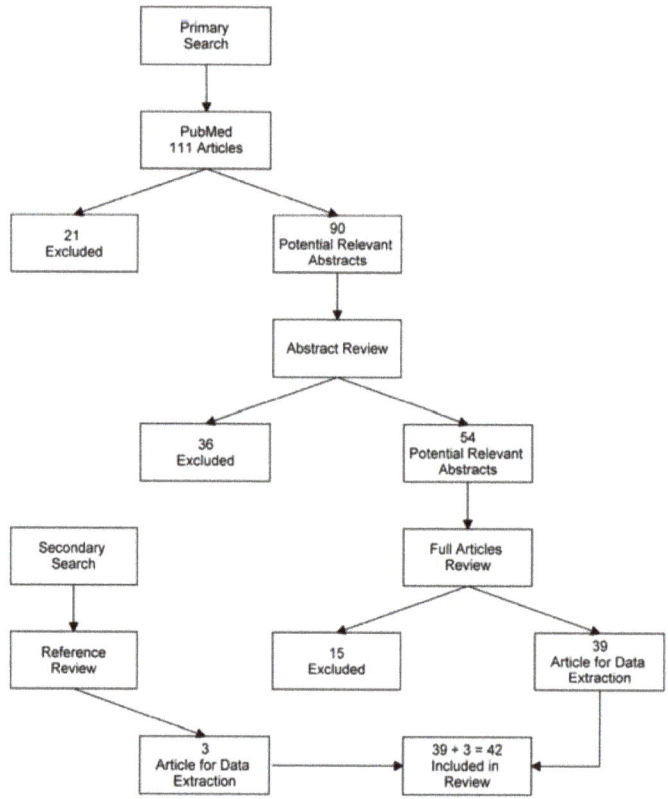

Figure A1. PRISMA flow diagram.

References

1. Sonfield, A.; Hasstedt, K.; Kavanaugh, M.L.; Anderson, R. *The Social and Economic Benefits of Women's Ability to Determine Whether and When to Have Children*; Guttmacher Institute: New York, NY, USA, 2013.
2. Apter, D. Contraception options: Aspects unique to adolescent and young adult. *Best Pr. Res. Clin. Obstet. Gynaecol.* **2018**, *48*, 115–127. [CrossRef] [PubMed]
3. Elaut, E.; Buysse, A.; de Sutter, P.; Gerris, J.; de Cuypere, G.; T'Sjoen, G. Cycle-Related Changes in Mood, Sexual Desire, and Sexual Activity in Oral Contraception-Using and Nonhormonal-Contraception-Using Couples. *J. Sex Res.* **2016**, *53*, 125–136. [CrossRef] [PubMed]
4. Caruso, S.; Agnello, C.; Malandrino, C.; Presti, L.L.; Cicero, C.; Cianci, S. Do Hormones Influence Women's Sex? Sexual Activity over the Menstrual Cycle. *J. Sex. Med.* **2014**, *11*, 211–221. [CrossRef] [PubMed]
5. Kennedy, T.G.; Armstrong, D.T. Induction of vaginal mucification in rats with testosterone and 17β-hydroxy-5α-androstan-3-one. *Steroids* **1976**, *27*, 423–430. [CrossRef]
6. Traish, A.M.; Vignozzi, L.; Simon, J.A.; Goldstein, I.; Kim, N.N. Role of Androgens in Female Genitourinary Tissue Structure and Function: Implications in the Genitourinary Syndrome of Menopause. *Sex. Med. Rev.* **2018**, *6*, 558–571. [CrossRef] [PubMed]
7. Goldstein, A.T.; Belkin, Z.R.; Krapf, J.M.; Song, W.; Khera, M.; Jutrzonka, S.L.; Kim, N.N.; Burrows, L.J.; Goldstein, I. Polymorphisms of the androgen receptor gene and hormonal contraceptive induced provoked vestibulodynia. *J. Sex. Med.* **2014**, *11*, 2764–2771. [CrossRef]
8. Curlin, M.; Bursac, D. Cervical mucus: From biochemical structure to clinical implications. *Front. Biosci.* **2013**, *5*, 507–515. [CrossRef]
9. Basson, R. Human sexual response. *Handb. Clin. Neurol.* **2015**, *130*, 11–18.
10. Davis, A.R.; Castaño, P.M. Oral contraceptives and libido in women. *Annu. Rev. Sex Res.* **2004**, *15*, 297–320.

11. Dobbins, J.G. Implication of a time-dependent model of sexual intercourse within the menstrual cycle. *J. Biosoc. Sci.* **1980**, *12*, 133–140. [CrossRef]
12. Burrows, L.J.; Basha, M.; Goldstein, A.T. The Effects of Hormonal Contraceptives on Female Sexuality: A Review. *J. Sex. Med.* **2012**, *9*, 2213–2223. [CrossRef]
13. Caruso, S.; Rugolo, S.; Agnello, C.; Romano, M.; Cianci, A. Quality of Sexual Life in Hyperandrogenic Women Treated with an Oral Contraceptive Containing Chlormadinone Acetate. *J. Sex. Med.* **2009**, *6*, 3376–3384. [CrossRef]
14. Both, S.; Lew-Starowicz, M.; Luria, M.; Sartorius, G.; Maseroli, E.; Tripodi, F.; Lowenstein, L.; Nappi, R.E.; Corona, G.; Reisman, Y.; et al. Hormonal Contraception and Female Sexuality: Position Statements from the European Society of Sexual Medicine (ESSM). *J. Sex. Med.* **2019**, *16*, 1681–1695. [CrossRef]
15. Casado-Espada, N.M.; de Alarcón, R.; de La Iglesia-Larrad, J.I.; Bote-Bonaechea, B.; Montejo, Á.L. Hormonal Contraceptives, Female Sexual Dysfunction, and Managing Strategies: A Review. *J. Clin. Med.* **2019**, *8*, 908. [CrossRef]
16. Shifren, J.L. The Role of Androgens in Female Sexual Dysfunction. *Mayo Clin. Proc.* **2004**, *79*, S19–S24. [CrossRef]
17. Toit, R.L.-D.; Perkins, M.S.; Hapgood, J.P.; Africander, D. Comparing the androgenic and estrogenic properties of progestins used in contraception and hormone therapy. *Biochem. Biophys. Res. Commun.* **2017**, *491*, 140–146. [CrossRef]
18. Caruso, S.; Malandrino, C.; Cicero, C.; Ciancio, F.; Cariola, M.; Cianci, A. Quality of Sexual Life of Women on Oral Contraceptive Continued-Regimen: Pilot Study. *J. Sex. Med.* **2013**, *10*, 460–466. [CrossRef]
19. Kuhl, H. Pharmacology of estrogens and progestogens: Influence of different routes of administration. *Climacteric* **2005**, *8*, 3–63. [CrossRef]
20. Di Carlo, C.; Gargano, V.; Sparice, S.; Tommaselli, G.A.; Bifulco, G.; Nappi, C. Effects of an oral contraceptive containing estradiol valerate and dienogest on circulating androgen levels and acne in young patients with PCOS: An observational preliminary study. *Gynecol. Endocrinol.* **2013**, *29*, 1048–1050. [CrossRef]
21. Caruso, S.; Cianci, S.; Cariola, M.; Fava, V.; di Pasqua, S.; Cianci, A. Improvement of Low Sexual Desire Due to Antiandrogenic Combined Oral Contraceptives After Switching to an Oral Contraceptive Containing 17β-Estradiol. *J. Women's Health* **2017**, *26*, 728–734. [CrossRef]
22. De Leo, V.; di Sabatino, A.; Musacchio, M.C.; Morgante, G.; Scolaro, V.; Cianci, A.; Petraglia, F. Effect of oral contraceptives on markers of hyperandrogenism and SHBG in women with polycystic ovary syndrome. *Contraception* **2010**, *82*, 276–280. [CrossRef]
23. Davis, S.R.; Bitzer, J.; Giraldi, A.; Palacios, S.; Parke, S.; Serrani, M.; Mellinger, U.; Nappi, R.E. Change to either a nonandrogenic or androgenic progestin-containing oral contraceptive preparation is associated with improved sexual function in women with oral contraceptive-associated sexual dysfunction. *J. Sex. Med.* **2013**, *10*, 3069–3079. [CrossRef]
24. Caruso, S.; Agnello, C.; Romano, M.; Cianci, S.; Presti, L.L.; Malandrino, C.; Cianci, A. Preliminary study on the effect of four-phasic estradiol valerate and dienogest (E2V/DNG) oral contraceptive on the quality of sexual life. *J. Sex. Med.* **2011**, *8*, 2841–2850. [CrossRef]
25. Burrows, L.J.; Goldstein, A.T. The Treatment of Vestibulodynia with Topical Estradiol and Testosterone. *Sex. Med.* **2013**, *1*, 30–33. [CrossRef]
26. Smith, N.K.; Jozkowski, K.N.; Sanders, S.A. Hormonal Contraception and Female Pain, Orgasm and Sexual Pleasure. *J. Sex. Med.* **2014**, *11*, 462–470. [CrossRef]
27. Caruso, S.; Agnello, C.; Intelisano, G.; Farina, M.; di Mari, L.; Cianci, A. Sexual behavior of women taking low-dose oral contraceptive containing 15 μg ethinylestradiol/60 μg gestodene. *Contraception* **2004**, *69*, 237–240. [CrossRef]
28. Pastor, Z.; Holla, K.; Chmel, R. The influence of combined oral contraceptives on female sexual desire: A systematic review. *Eur. J. Contracept. Reprod. Health Care* **2013**, *18*, 27–43. [CrossRef]
29. Graham, C.A.; Bancroft, J.; Doll, H.A.; Greco, T.; Tanner, A. Does oral contraceptive-induced reduction in free testosterone adversely affect the sexuality or mood of women? *Psychoneuroendocrinology* **2007**, *32*, 246–255. [CrossRef] [PubMed]
30. Wallwiener, C.W.; Wallwiener, L.-M.; Seeger, H.; Schönfisch, B.; Mueck, A.O.; Bitzer, J.; Zipfel, S.; Brucker, S.Y.; Taran, F.-A.; Wallwiener, M. Are hormonal components of oral contraceptives associated with impaired female sexual function? A questionnaire-based online survey of medical students in Germany, Austria, and Switzerland. *Arch. Gynecol. Obstet.* **2015**, *292*, 883–890. [CrossRef] [PubMed]
31. Bancroft, J.; Hammond, G.; Graham, C. Do oral contraceptives produce irreversible effects on women's sexuality? *J. Sex. Med.* **2006**, *3*, 567. [CrossRef] [PubMed]
32. Serati, M.; Bogani, G.; di Dedda, M.C.; Braghiroli, A.; Uccella, S.; Cromi, A.; Ghezzi, F. A comparison between vaginal estrogen and vaginal hyaluronic for the treatment of dyspareunia in women using hormonal contraceptive. *Eur. J. Obstet. Gynecol. Reprod. Biol.* **2015**, *191*, 48–50. [CrossRef]
33. Caruso, S.; Panella, M.; Giunta, G.; Matarazzo, M.G.; Cianci, A.; Cianci, S. Comparative randomized study on the sexual function and quality of life of women on contraceptive vaginal ring containing ethinylestradiol/etonogestrel 3.47/11.00 mg or 2.7/11.7 mg. *Gynecol. Endocrinol.* **2019**, *35*, 1–5. [CrossRef]
34. Guida, M.; di Carlo, C.; Troisi, J.; Gallo, A.; Cibarelli, F.; Martini, E.; Tiranini, L.; Nappi, R.E. The sexuological impact of hormonal contraceptives based on their route of administration. *Gynecol. Endocrinol.* **2017**, *33*, 218–222. [CrossRef]
35. Elaut, E.; Buysse, A.; de Sutter, P.; de Cuypere, G.; Gerris, J.; Deschepper, E.; T'Sjoen, G. Relation of androgen receptor sensitivity and mood to sexual desire in hormonal contraception users. *Contraception* **2012**, *85*, 470–479. [CrossRef]

36. Caruso, S.; Cianci, S.; Malandrino, C.; Cicero, C.; Presti, L.L.; Cianci, A. Quality of sexual life of women using the contraceptive vaginal ring in extended cycles: Preliminary report. *Eur. J. Contracept. Reprod. Health Care* **2014**, *19*, 307–314. [CrossRef]
37. Mohamed, A.M.M.; El-Sherbiny, W.S.M.; Mostafa, W.A.I. Combined contraceptive ring versus combined oral contraceptive (30 µg ethinylestradiol and 3-mg drospirenone). *Int. J. Gynecol. Obstet.* **2011**, *114*, 145–148. [CrossRef]
38. Department of Reproductive Health; World Health Organization. *Medical Eligibility Criteria for Contraceptive Use*, 4th ed.; World Health Organization: Geneva, Switzerland, 2010.
39. Gracia, C.R.; Sammel, M.D.; Charlesworth, S.; Lin, H.; Barnhart, K.T.; Creinin, M.D. Sexual function in first-time contraceptive ring and contraceptive patch users. *Fertil. Steril.* **2010**, *93*, 21–28. [CrossRef]
40. Graham, C.A.; Ramos, R.; Bancroft, J.; Maglaya, C.; Farley, T.M. The effects of steroidal contraceptives on the well-being and sexuality of women: A double-blind, placebo-controlled, two-centre study of combined and progestogen-only methods. *Contraception* **1995**, *52*, 363–369. [CrossRef]
41. McCoy, N.L.; Matyas, J.R. Oral contraceptives and sexuality in university women. *Arch. Sex. Behav.* **1996**, *25*, 73–90. [CrossRef]
42. Jung-Hoffman, C.; Kuhl, H. Divergent effects of two low-dose oral contraceptives on sex hormone-binding globulin and free testosterone. *Am. J. Obstet. Gynecol.* **1987**, *156*, 199–203. [CrossRef]
43. Secura, G.M.; Allsworth, J.E.; Madden, T.; Mullersman, J.L.; Peipert, J.F. The Contraceptive CHOICE Project: Reducing barriers to long-acting reversible contraception. *Am. J. Obstet. Gynecol.* **2010**, *203*, 115.e1–115.e7. [CrossRef]
44. Rose, S.B.; Lawton, B.A. Impact of long-acting reversible contraception on return for repeat abortion. *Am. J. Obstet. Gynecol.* **2012**, *206*, 37.e1–e6. [CrossRef] [PubMed]
45. Grunloh, D.S.; Casner, T.; Secura, G.M.; Peipert, J.F.; Madden, T.S.D. Characteristics Associated With Discontinuation of Long-Acting Reversible Contraception Within the First 6 Months of Use. *Obstet. Gynecol.* **2013**, *122*, 1214–1221. [CrossRef] [PubMed]
46. Sanders, J.N.; Higgins, J.A.; Adkins, D.E.; Stoddard, G.J.; Gawron, L.M.; Turok, D.K. The Impact of Sexual Satisfaction, Functioning, and Perceived Contraceptive Effects on Sex Life on IUD and Implant Continuation at 1 Year. *Women's Health Issues* **2018**, *28*, 401–407. [CrossRef] [PubMed]
47. Gomez, A.M.; Clark, J.B. The relationship between contraceptive features preferred by young women and interest in IUDs: An exploratory analysis. *Perspect. Sex. Reprod. Health* **2014**, *46*, 157–163. [CrossRef]
48. Neri, M.; Piras, B.; Paoletti, A.M.; Vallerino, V.; Corda, V.; Ronchetti, C.; Taccori, V.; Pilloni, M.; Zedda, P.; Capobianco, G.; et al. Long-acting reversible contraception (LARC) with the intrauterine system with levonorgestrel (6mcg/d): Observational study on the acceptability, quality of life, and sexuality in Italian women. *Gynecol. Endocrinol.* **2018**, *34*, 532–535. [CrossRef] [PubMed]
49. Caruso, S.; Cianci, S.; Vitale, S.G.; Fava, V.; Cutello, S.; Cianci, A. Sexual function and quality of life of women adopting the levonorgestrel-releasing intrauterine system (LNG-IUS 13.5 mg) after abortion for unintended pregnancy. *Eur. J. Contracept. Reprod. Health Care* **2018**, *23*, 24–31. [CrossRef]
50. Higgins, J.A.; Kramer, R.D.; Wright, K.Q.; Everett, B.; Turok, D.K.; Sanders, J.N. Sexual Functioning, Satisfaction, and Well-Being Among Contraceptive Users: A Three-Month Assessment From the HER Salt Lake Contraceptive Initiative. *J. Sex Res.* **2021**, *9*, 1–10. [CrossRef]
51. Higgins, J.A.; Ryder, K.; Skarda, G.; Koepsel, E.; Bennett, E.A. The Sexual Acceptability of Intrauterine Contraception: A Qualitative Study of Young Adult Women. *Perspect. Sex. Reprod. Health* **2015**, *47*, 115–122. [CrossRef]
52. Pekin, A.T.; Kerimoğlu, O.S.; Kebapcılar, A.G.; Yılmaz, S.A.; Benzer, N.; Celik, C. Depressive symptomatology and quality of life assessment among women using the levonorgestrel-releasing intrauterine system: An observational study. *Arch. Gynecol. Obstet.* **2014**, *290*, 507–511. [CrossRef]
53. Higgins, J.A.; Smith, N.K. The Sexual Acceptability of Contraception: Reviewing the Literature and Building a New Concept. *J. Sex Res.* **2016**, *53*, 417–456. [CrossRef]
54. Enzlin, P.; Weyers, S.; Janssens, D.; Poppe, W.; Eelen, C.; Pazmany, E.; Elaut, E.; Amy, J. Sexual Functioning in Women Using Levonorgestrel-Releasing Intrauterine Systems as Compared to Copper Intrauterine Devices. *J. Sex. Med.* **2012**, *9*, 1065–1073. [CrossRef]
55. Malmborg, A.; Brynhildsen, J.; Hammar, M. A survey of young women's perceptions of the influence of the Levonorgestrel-Intrauterine System or copper-intrauterine device on sexual desire. *Sex. Reprod. Health* **2019**, *21*, 75–80. [CrossRef]
56. He, Y.R.; Li, Y.; Ma, L.; Wei, S.S.; Wu, H.Y.; Huang, J. Effects of LNG-IUS on sexual function and sexual quality in women of childbearing age. *Zhonghua Yi Xue Za Zhi* **2020**, *100*, 1255–1259.
57. Ferreira, J.M.; Carreiro, A.V.; Fernandes, A.; Bahamondes, L. Sexual Function and Quality of Life in a Cohort of Brazilian Users of Two Kind of Intrauterine Contraceptives. *Rev. Bras. Ginecol. Obstet.* **2019**, *41*, 236–241. [CrossRef]
58. Apter, D. International Perspectives: IUDs and Adolescents. *J. Pediatr. Adolesc. Gynecol.* **2019**, *32*, S36–S42. [CrossRef]
59. Caruso, S.; Vitale, S.G.; Fava, V.; di Pasqua, S.; Rapisarda, A.M.C.; Cianci, S. Quality of life of women using the etonogestrel long-acting reversible contraceptive implant after abortion for unplanned pregnancy. *Eur. J. Contracept. Reprod. Health Care* **2020**, *25*, 251–258. [CrossRef]
60. Walsh-Buhi, E.R.; Helmy, H.L. Trends in long-acting reversible contraceptive (LARC) use, LARC use predictors, and dual-method use among a national sample of college women. *J. Am. Coll. Health* **2018**, *66*, 225–236. [CrossRef]
61. Di Carlo, C.; Sansone, A.; de Rosa, N.; Gargano, V.; Tommaselli, G.A.; Nappi, C.; Bifulco, G. Impact of an implantable steroid contraceptive (etonogestrel-releasing implant) on quality of life and sexual function: A preliminary study. *Gynecol. Endocrinol.* **2014**, *30*, 53–56. [CrossRef]

62. Higgins, J.A.; Hirsch, J.S. Pleasure, Power, and Inequality: Incorporating Sexuality into Research on Contraceptive Use. *Am. J. Public Health* **2008**, *98*, 1803–1813. [CrossRef]
63. Fennell, J. "And Isn't that the point?": Pleasure and contraceptive decisions. *Contraception* **2014**, *89*, 264–270. [CrossRef] [PubMed]
64. Lu, C.F.; Vargas, S.E.; Guillen, M.; Ramirez, J.J.; Carbone, S.L.; Getz, M.L.; Frimpong, Y.; Smith, K.A.; Shaw, J.G.; Tong, I.; et al. A Qualitative Study of the Contraceptive Effect on Women's Sexual Experiences: Beyond Hormonal Effects. *Obstet. Gynecol.* **2019**, *134*, 91–101. [CrossRef] [PubMed]
65. Stuckey, B.G. Female Sexual Function and Dysfunction in the Reproductive Years: The Influence of Endogenous and Exogenous Sex Hormones. *J. Sex. Med.* **2008**, *5*, 2282–2290. [CrossRef] [PubMed]

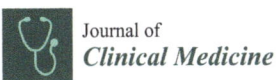

Article

Long-Acting Reversible Contraception: Placement, Continuation, and Removal Rates at an Inner-City Academic Medical Center Clinic

Aliye Runyan [1], Robert A. Welch [2], Katherine J. Kramer [3], Sarah Cortez [4], LeAnne J. Roberts [4], Clementina Asamoah [4], Sarah Ottum [5], Jessica Sanders [6], Adib Shafi [7] and Maurice-Andre Recanati [8,*]

1. Department of Obstetrics and Gynecology, Westchester Medical Center, Valhalla, NY 10595, USA; alrunyan@gmail.com
2. Department of Obstetrics and Gynecology, Hurley Medical Center, Flint, MI 48503, USA; rwelch2@hurleymc.com
3. Department of Obstetrics and Gynecology, St. Vincent's Catholic Medical Centers, New York, NY 10011, USA; katherinekramer@gmail.com
4. Department of Obstetrics and Gynecology, Wayne State University, Detroit, MI 48202, USA; sarah.cortez@wayne.edu (S.C.); lroberts@med.wayne.edu (L.J.R.); asamoahc@gmail.com (C.A.)
5. Department of Surgery, Wayne State University, Detroit, MI 48202, USA; Sottum@med.wayne.edu
6. Department of Obstetrics and Gynecology, University of Utah, Salt Lake City, UT 84132, USA; jessica.sanders@hsc.utah.edu
7. Department of Computer Science, Wayne State University, Detroit, MI 48202, USA; fj9079@wayne.edu
8. NIH-Women's Reproductive Health Research (WRHR) Scholar, Department of Obstetrics and Gynecology, Wayne State University, Detroit, MI 48202, USA
* Correspondence: marecanati@wayne.edu

Abstract: Long-Acting Reversible Contraception (LARCs) has the potential to decrease unintended pregnancies but only if women can easily access a requested method. Retrospective electronic chart review identified women desiring LARC placement over a one-year period ending 31 December 2016. Most of the 311 insertions were for family planning, with 220 new insertions and 60 replacements. Delays occurred in 38% ($n = 118$) of patients, averaged 5 ± 5 weeks, and 47% received interval contraception. Reasons included absence of qualified provider ($n = 44$, 37%), pending cultures ($n = 31$, 26%), and Mirena availability. Teenage LARC use favored Nexplanon whereas older women preferred Mirena ($p < 0.01$). Of the 11% choosing early LARC removal, a significant number were African Americans ($p = 0.040$) or teenagers ($p = 0.048$). Retention time varied by device type; most patients switched to other contraceptives. No patients experienced IUD expulsion. Understanding barriers, attempting to remedy them, and addressing the side effects associated with LARC use is of importance in this inner-city patient population in the United States.

Keywords: long-acting reversible contraception; intrauterine device; LARC placement delays; removal rates; inner-city clinic

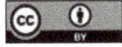

1. Introduction

About six million pregnancies occur yearly in the United States, with approximately 45–51% of these unintended [1]. Compared to other industrialized nations, this rate is substantially higher [2], and worldwide 44% of pregnancies are unintended, with rates as high as 65% in developing nations [3]. Although unintended pregnancies affect all women, rates were disproportionately highest among those who were cohabitating, below the poverty line or were non-Hispanic Blacks [1]. About 54% experiencing unintended pregnancy reported using contraception at the time they conceived [4]. Inconsistent method use accounts for 90% of these pregnancies rather than method failure (10%) [5]. About 25% of at-risk women experience one or more months with a gap in contraceptive use [6]. Lack of college education, ambivalence about pregnancy, being Black, being 35–44 years of age, method-related difficulties, side effects and dissatisfaction with the current method were strongly associated with inconsistent contraceptive use [7].

Of the 61 million U.S. women aged 14–44 years old, 61.7% are currently using contraception [8]. Common methods include oral contraceptives (16–38%), male condoms (9.4–32%), long-acting reversible contraceptives (LARC) (7.2–12%), and female sterilization (15.5–25%) [5,9]. These rates are comparable with other nations such as Europe (10–32%) and Australia (7%) [10]. Failure rates in the first year are 9%, 18%, 0.05–0.8%, and 0.1–0.8%, respectively [11]. Reasons for inconsistent use of user-dependent methods include absence from home, depletion of supplies, illness, lack of inclination, perception of being at low risk for pregnancy, attitudes about pregnancy, and experiences with unintended pregnancy [4,5].

LARC methods of contraception are highly effective yet may be underused [11]. Only about 12% of women currently employ LARC contraception, of whom 10% use intrauterine devices (IUDs) while 1.3% have subdermal implants (SDIs) [9]. Barriers to LARC utilization include patient lack of knowledge [12], bias in counselling by healthcare providers [13,14], lack of provider training and competency [15], and the up-front cost of these devices [16]. When patients are well educated, and when costs are not a factor, such as for female OBGYN residents, 53% chose LARC methods [17]. Similarly, for patients enrolled in the CHOICE Project, which provided education and no-cost birth control, a majority of women (67%) choose LARCs [18]. Because LARC methods are "forgettable," effectiveness is user-independent, and they eliminate the common shortfalls previously described for other contraceptives. LARCs have some of the highest rates of continuation after one year—84% for Implanon [11] and greater than 80% for IUDs [11]—with patient satisfaction rates mirroring continuation rates [19,20]. These devices have been shown to be safe [21] and effective in all women regardless of parity [22] and their use has been increasing in younger women [23].

In order to prevent unintended pregnancies and their associated financial [24] and social [25] costs, effective contraceptives, such as LARCs, must be readily accessible and barriers to insertion minimized. Since nearly half of patients intending to use an IUD failed to return for placement during a subsequent visit [26], single visit protocols ensure that more women have access to contraception in a timely manner. The insurance restriction of combining a well-woman exam with IUD insertion, the availability of the device, and pre-insertion screening all may cause such delays. Multiple studies have shown that in women with asymptomatic sexually transmitted diseases, IUD placement did not increase the risk of pelvic inflammatory disease (PID) [27,28]. Thus, screening can be done at the time of insertion and treatment given subsequently [29].

For a contraceptive to be effective it must be continuously used, yet a minority of patients opt to discontinue their method for reasons other than planning pregnancy [30]. Common adverse effects of LARCs include abnormal bleeding, amenorrhea, dysmenorrhea, pelvic pain [31] and, for implants, rod migration, mood swings, and headaches [32]. While LARCs are FDA approved to remain in place for 3 to 10 years, women who experience intolerable side effects may opt for "early" removal [33–35]. Many patients requesting removal of LARCs also complained of a lack of disclosure of all possible side effects and encountered delays after they requested removal, raising concerns about provider's attitudes and respect for body autonomy [36,37].

LARC utilization patterns at the downtown campus of the Detroit Medical Center are likely to reflect those of other large urban populations. Little is known, however, about LARC acceptance by underserved women in the impersonal environment of such large urban medical centers that are staffed by resident physicians and nurse practitioners. The impact of high-volume clinic care on the acceptance of LARCs may have significant population health implications. The purpose of this study was to evaluate LARC utilization in the setting of a large urban academic center.

2. Materials and Methods

Patient Selection

Under IRB approval (WSU 074517MP2E), a retrospective electronic health record (EHR) review was performed to identify women who requested LARC placement in the resident clinic for a one-year period from 1 January through 31 December 2016. Included were non-pregnant women [38] desiring LARC contraception. IUDs (Mirena and Paragard) and implants (Nexplanon) were analyzed separately. Information from each patient included: demographic data, prior contraceptive method, proximity to previous childbirth, date of LARC request, date of LARC placement, type of device, provider (resident, physician or nurse practitioner), reason device was inserted (e.g., family planning, replace expiring device, abnormal bleeding) and an explanation for delays, defined as failure to place a device at the initial visit. Records were reviewed for prescription of bridging contraceptive methods during this delay period. Patients receiving LARCs during the study period were followed for an additional year to identify those requesting early LARC removal, the date of this request, reason, and actual date the device was removed, as well as their new contraceptive method, if any.

Quantile-quantile plots were used to examine normality of numeric variables. Median differences were examined using the Kruskal–Wallis or Mann–Whitney U tests, as appropriate. Differences in proportions were tested using the Fisher's exact test, as appropriate. We used logistic regression to examine magnitudes of association adjusting for potentially confounding factors. Statistical significance was considered to be $p < 0.05$ or 95% confidence interval (CI), not including the null estimate of association (i.e., odds ratio (OR) = 1.0).

3. Results

This study included 311 participants. LARC device utilization by age and ethnicity is shown in Table 1.

Table 1. Utilization of Long-Acting Reversible Contraception by Age and Ethnicity.

	N (%)	Mirena	Paragard	Nexplanon
Average Age (±SD)	28.2 (±7.9)	30.9 (±7.6)	28.4 (±7.4)	24.1 (±6.8)
Age range	13–51	14–51	17–46	13–44
African American	266 (85)	146	18	102
Middle Eastern	18 (6)	3	14	1
Asian	15 (5)	2	13	0
White	10 (3)	5	2	3
Hispanic	2 (<1)	1	0	1
Family Planning—New device insertions	220 (71)	90	43	87
Family Planning—Replacement of expired device	60 (19)	36	4	20
Abnormal Uterine Bleeding	31 (10)	31	0	0
Total	311 (100)	157	47	107

3.1. Indication for Device Placement

The majority of LARCs were placed for family planning indications ($n = 280$) with $n = 220$ new device insertions and $n = 60$ replacement of an expired device. A significant number of new devices placed included Nexplanon and Paragard ($n = 87$, $p < 0.004$; and $n = 43$, $p < 0.001$, respectively), compared to all insertions. A significant number of new family planning insertions were requested by Middle Eastern women ($n = 17$, $p = 0.014$), compared to all insertions for the indication of family planning. Abnormal uterine bleeding accounted for the remainder of insertions ($n = 31$), all of which were Mirena.

3.2. Device Distribution by Race

Across all cases (new insertions and replacements), Mirena was the most frequently chosen LARC ($n = 157$, 50%), followed by Nexplanon ($n = 107$, 34%) and Paragard ($n = 47$, 15%) as shown in Figure 1. African Americans chose Mirena significantly more than did the other races (Middle Eastern, Asian, White and Hispanic), 55% vs. 24% (146/266 vs. 11/45, $p < 0.001$). Similarly, African Americans chose Nexplanon significantly more often than did the other races, 38% vs. 11% (102/266 vs. 5/45, $p < 0.001$). On the other hand, the other groups, particularly Middle Eastern, chose Paragard significantly more than did African Americans, 64% vs. just 7% (29/45 vs. 18/266, $p < 0.001$).

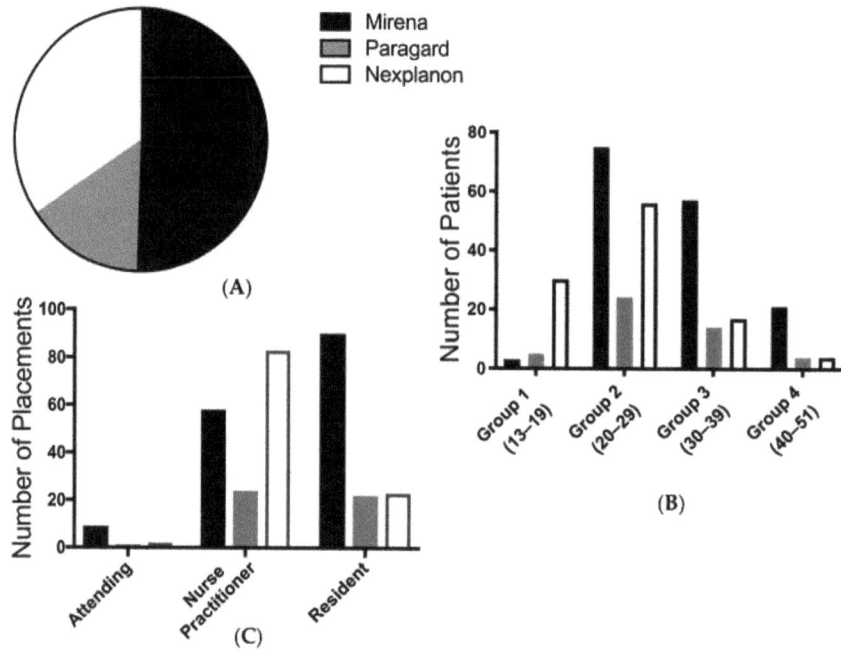

Figure 1. LARC devices placed in 2016 (**A**) by device type ($n = 311$); (**B**) by age group; (**C**) by provider type.

3.3. Device Distribution by Age

For analysis purposes, age ranges were divided into four groups: group 1: 13–19 years old ($n = 38$), group 2: 20–29 ($n = 155$), group 3: 30–39 ($n = 89$), group 4: 40–51 ($n = 29$). A significant number of patients from group 4 chose Mirena ($n = 21$, $p = 0.01$), while a significant number of teenagers chose Nexplanon ($n = 30$, $p < 0.001$), as shown in Figure 1.

3.4. Analysis of Delays in LARC Placement

Out of 311 patients, 38% (118) experienced delays requiring more than one visit for the placement of their LARC, and the mean length of the delay was 4.8 weeks ± 4.8 (SD, range 1 week to 7 months).

African American women were significantly more likely to experience a delay in LARC placement compared to other races taken as a whole (108/266 = 41% vs. 10/45 = 22%, $p = 0.020$). There was no significant difference, however, in the duration of delay by race.

Those choosing Mirena were significantly more likely to experience a delay in LARC placement compared to the other two devices taken as a whole (69/157 = 59% vs. 49/154 = 32%, $p = 0.035$). There was no significant difference, however, in the duration of delay by device.

Stated reasons for delaying LARC placement included absence of a qualified provider ($n = 44$, 37%), pending gonorrhea/chlamydial test results ($n = 31$, 26%), and reason unknown (n = 30, 25%), with the remainder consisting of scheduling issues (n = 2), recent intercourse (n = 2), abnormal pap (n = 1), unexplained vaginal bleeding (n = 1), pending endometrial biopsy (n = 4), retained IUD (n = 2) and uterine abnormality (n = 1) (Figure 2). A significant number of patients who were delayed for pending gonorrhea/chlamydial cultures had chosen Mirena compared to all who were delayed (p = 0.007, n = 25 of 31 compared to 69 of 118). Patients who chose Nexplanon had significantly less delay in placement (p = 0.020) when the device was inserted by residents (n = 8 of 35) as opposed to nurse practitioners (n = 26 of 35). No other association was found between the delay in LARC placement and the type of medical provider. No significant association was found between patient age and delay in LARC placement. Forty-seven percent of women experiencing delays were bridged with contraceptives including condoms (n = 24, 21%) or continuation of existing method (n = 29, 26%) such as Depo-Provera or IUD, while the rest were either not offered contraception or no documentation could be found.

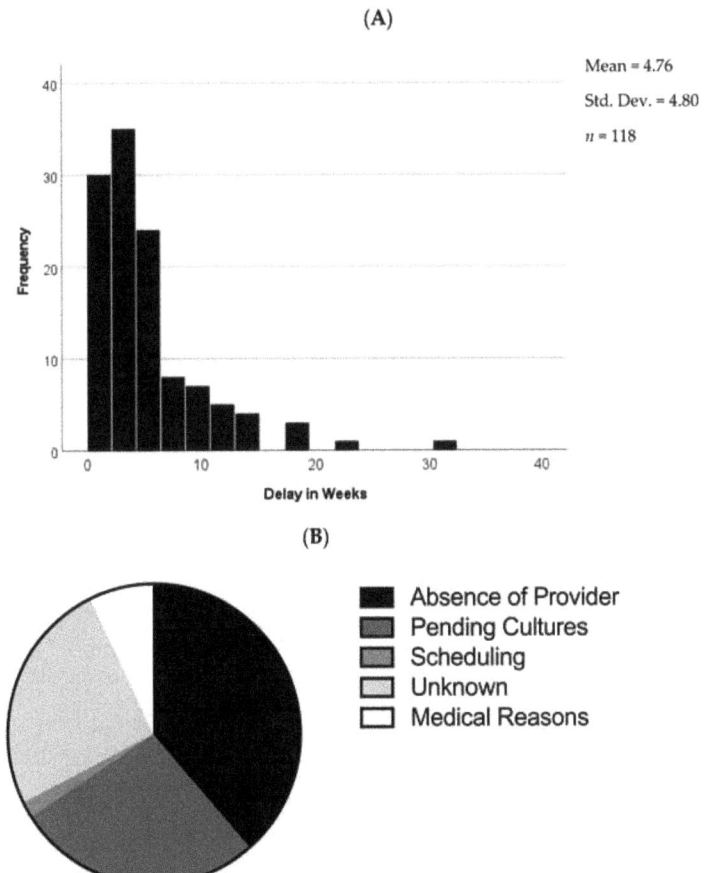

Figure 2. Delay in LARC Placement. (A) Length of delay; (B) reasons for delay.

3.5. Analysis of Device Removal

Thirty-four women chose to have their LARC device removed (17 Mirena, 16 Nexplanon, 1 Paragard). Out of this group, n = 24 (71%) were new insertions. The average length of retention for those who chose removal was 162 days (range 8–356 days) but varied significantly (p = 0.02) by device type: Mirena (4.2 months ± 2.8 SD) vs. Nexplanon

(6.8 months ± 3.2 SD) (Figure 3). No significant relation was found with the type of provider placing the device. Nearly all the women who chose to remove their LARC were African American (33/34, $p = 0.040$). A significant number who chose removal were teenagers ($n = 8$, $p = 0.048$). Only 3% (1 of 34, $p = 0.39$) discontinued Paragard, despite Paragard comprising 15% of all devices (47 of 311). No patients experienced IUD expulsion.

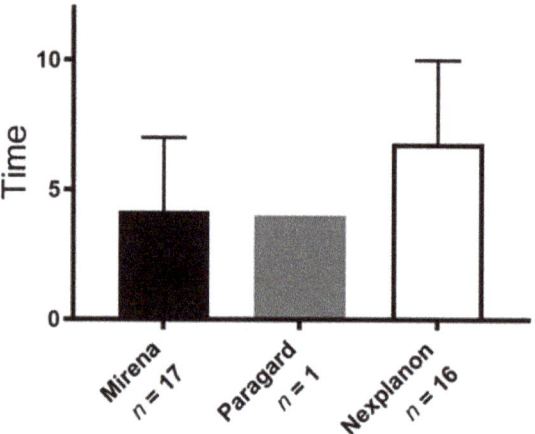

Figure 3. Thirty-four (11%) women chose early removal of their LARC. Mean time (in months) from insertion to removal varied significantly by device type. Error bars represent SD.

3.6. Analysis of Switching out of LARC Method

Of the 34 women who removed their LARC, twenty-four elected to switch to an alternate method of contraception. These included: OCPs ($n = 10$), depot-medroxyprogesterone acetate ($n = 9$), Paragard ($n = 1$), patch ($n = 1$), Mirena ($n = 1$), NuvaRing ($n = 1$), and barrier methods ($n = 1$). Of all age groups, teenagers were also most likely to switch to another form of birth control ($n = 8$, $p = 0.018$).

4. Discussion

4.1. Delay in Placement

The majority of LARC placements were for family planning and 21% (60/280) of placements consisted of replacement of an expiring device. Our experience in this urban clinic demonstrates that 38% of patients requesting LARC experienced significant delays in placement. Lack of provider education and particularly the belief that IUD placement requires knowledge of the results of gonorrhea/chlamydia testing [39], the absence of a qualified providers, and scheduling issues accounted for about two-thirds of these delays (Figure 2). Mirena was the most frequently chosen LARC, but women opting for this device experienced the greatest delays due to pending cultures ($p = 0.022$) and because of lack of device availability.

Unintended pregnancy remains a major public health issue [1]. LARC contraceptives, when placed on the day that the patient requests it, provides immediate protection from unintended pregnancy. In women where it is "reasonably certain" [38] that they are not pregnant, same day placement should be the goal [40]. When compared to patients requesting hormonal methods, 95% women (697/737) who met the criteria walked out with a prescription. These factors may be addressed through provider education and improved clinic management. Clinicians should offer bridging contraception to prevent pregnancy regardless of the reason for the delay in LARC placement.

4.2. Early Removal of Device

We found that both subdermal implants (SDI) and IUDs had high continuation rates (90%) and low numbers of complications in the first-year post-insertion, consistent with other studies [19,35,41]. These rates surpass those of short-acting contraceptives such as the patch (10%) and the pill (32%) [42]. Unlike other studies [41], we found that removal rates were not associated with type of provider placing the device. This may be due to the formal training clinicians practicing at our institution receive which ensures that patients universally receive adequate pre-placement counselling.

About 10% of LARCs in our study were inserted in teenagers, reflecting a growing acceptance of long-acting contraceptives in this age group [43]. Similar to other studies [33,44], we observed that SDIs were prescribed significantly more in teens. This may be due to an ongoing bias from less informed physicians on the use of IUDs in nulliparous patients [45], and in particularly teens [14]. This group also experienced a significantly higher number of complications, particularly spotting, but were most likely to switch to another form of birth control. Conversely, older women were more likely to opt for an IUD, particularly Mirena, as this method is also indicated for the treatment of abnormal uterine bleeding. Similar to other studies, we found that this age group tended to have high retention rates for their LARC [30]. Future studies may also examine the decision to choose LARCs over other methods where metabolic [46] and vascular effects, weight gain, body image [47] and sexual behavior [48] impact patient wellbeing.

Concerns involving early removal of LARCs go beyond the simple cost-effectiveness calculation and include risks of unintended pregnancies associated with no contraception or suboptimal protection. Frequently, patients present to clinic requesting removal of their device because of pain, changes in bleeding patterns, mood swings, weight gain or other reasons. Studies have shown that these women tended to reluctantly tolerate these side effects but eventually reached a tipping point [32]. A close follow up with patients who received LARCs may help ensure that clinicians can intervene in alleviating the side effects of the LARC. While some physicians tend to be reluctant to remove LARCs, it is critical that they respect patient autonomy and support a woman's decision-making around contraceptive use [36]. Teaching patients about IUD self-removal [49] could have a positive impact on reproductive autonomy. The effects of women seeking removal from other willing clinicians, or removing the device on their own, may influence the results of our study and will be examined by prospective trials in the future.

A strength of our study is the inclusion of African American women of all age ranges. The study was limited by using a single urban health clinic where the majority of patients had public health insurance [25]. Further study in different geographic areas or in women with private insurance may alter our findings or limit generalizability. If patients received care for LARC-related issues at other clinics, or lost Medicaid eligibility, continuation rates may be falsely high. While the electronic health record (EHR) was used to access contraception encounter data, the accuracy of the records has the potential for incomplete data [50], which may affect results. One such limitation is the inability of our EHR to ascertain the number of women who intended to be on LARC but were unable to obtain it and never returned.

5. Conclusions

Although the American College of Obstetrics and Gynecology recommends same-day LARC placement in eligible patients, this study elucidates some of the challenges encountered in making same-day insertion practical in a large urban clinic. Realizing that women requesting family planning visits should be considered urgent appointments can help protect women from undesired pregnancy. Controlling device inventory, having trained providers present and educating on latest guidelines are necessary to fulfill patient expectations. In all circumstances, clinicians must offer the patient a reliable means of contraception in the interim. Reasons why women chose LARC removal and choose other, less reliable forms of contraception need further study.

Author Contributions: Conceptualization, A.R. and M.-A.R.; methodology, K.J.K. and S.C.; software, S.O., J.S. and A.S.; validation, S.O., J.S. and S.O.; formal analysis, A.S. and S.O.; investigation, L.J.R.; resources, S.C. and R.A.W.; data curation, S.O.; writing—original draft preparation, M.-A.R., R.A.W. and K.J.K.; writing—review and editing, R.A.W. and A.R.; visualization, C.A.; supervision, M.-A.R.; project administration, K.J.K.; funding acquisition, M.-A.R. All authors have read and agreed to the published version of the manuscript.

Funding: This research was supported under NIH-Women's Reproductive Health Research Career Development Award (K-12HD001254).

Institutional Review Board Statement: The Wayne State University Institutional Review Board approved IRB# 074517MP2E, LARC Placement, Continuation and Removal Rates in the DMC Ob-Gyn clinics (Protocol # 1707000720).

Informed Consent Statement: This is a retrospective chart review. All data was de-identified and informed consent was waved by the IRB.

Data Availability Statement: The datasets that support the findings of this study are available from the corresponding author (M.-A.R.) upon reasonable written request.

Acknowledgments: This research was made possible by the work and dedication of all the obstetrics and gynecology residents at Wayne State University and by the faculty and staff at the Detroit Medical Center. In particular, the Sorin Draghichi laboratory helped provide statistical analysis. We also wish to thank the NIH-Women's Reproductive Health Research Career Development Award at Wayne State University for ongoing research and support.

Conflicts of Interest: The authors declare no conflict of interest.

References

1. Finer, L.B.; Zolna, M.R. Declines in Unintended Pregnancy in the United States, 2008–2011. *N. Engl. J. Med.* **2016**, *374*, 843–852. [CrossRef] [PubMed]
2. Sedgh, G.; Singh, S.; Hussain, R. Intended and unintended pregnancies worldwide in 2012 and recent trends. *Stud. Fam. Plan.* **2014**, *45*, 301–314. [CrossRef] [PubMed]
3. Bearak, J.; Popinchalk, A.; Alkema, L.; Sedgh, G. Global, regional, and subregional trends in unintended pregnancy and its outcomes from 1990 to 2014: Estimates from a Bayesian hierarchical model. *Lancet Glob. Health* **2018**, *6*, e380–e389. [CrossRef]
4. Jones, R.K.; Darroch, J.E.; Henshaw, S.K. Contraceptive use among U.S. women having abortions in 2000–2001. *Perspect. Sex. Reprod. Health* **2002**, *34*, 294–303. [CrossRef] [PubMed]
5. Frost, J.J.; Darroch, J.E. Factors associated with contraceptive choice and inconsistent method use, United States, 2004. *Perspect. Sex. Reprod. Health* **2008**, *40*, 94–104. [CrossRef] [PubMed]
6. Frost, J.J.; Singh, S.; Finer, L.B. U.S. women's one-year contraceptive use patterns, 2004. *Perspect. Sex. Reprod. Health* **2007**, *39*, 48–55. [CrossRef] [PubMed]
7. Frost, J.J.; Singh, S.; Finer, L.B. Factors associated with contraceptive use and nonuse, United States, 2004. *Perspect. Sex. Reprod. Health* **2007**, *39*, 90–99. [CrossRef] [PubMed]
8. Daniels, K.; Mosher, W.D. *Contraceptive Methods Women Have Ever Used: United States, 1982–2010*; National Health Statistics Report; National Center for Health Statistics: Hyattsville, MD, USA, 2013; pp. 1–15.
9. Daniels, K.; Daugherty, J.; Jones, J. *Current Contraceptive Status among Women Aged 15–44: United States, 2011–2013*; NCHS Data Brief; National Center for Health Statistics: Hyattsville, MD, USA, 2014; pp. 1–8.
10. Eeckhaut, M.C.; Sweeney, M.M.; Gipson, J.D. Who is using long-acting reversible contraceptive methods? Findings from nine low-fertility countries. *Perspect. Sex. Reprod. Health* **2014**, *46*, 149–155. [CrossRef]
11. Trussell, J. Contraceptive failure in the United States. *Contraception* **2011**, *83*, 397–404. [CrossRef]
12. Forrest, J.D. U.S. women's perceptions of and attitudes about the IUD. *Obstet. Gynecol. Surv.* **1996**, *51*, S30–S34. [CrossRef]
13. Madden, T.; Allsworth, J.E.; Hladky, K.J.; Secura, G.M.; Peipert, J.F. Intrauterine contraception in Saint Louis: A survey of obstetrician and gynecologists' knowledge and attitudes. *Contraception* **2010**, *81*, 112–116. [CrossRef]
14. Diaz, V.A.; Hughes, N.; Dickerson, L.M.; Wessell, A.M.; Carek, P.J. Clinician knowledge about use of intrauterine devices in adolescents in South Carolina AHEC. *Fam. Med.* **2011**, *43*, 407–411.
15. Phillips, J.; Sandhu, P. Barriers to implementation of long-acting reversible contraception: A systematic review. *J. Am. Assoc. Nurse Pract.* **2018**, *30*, 236–243. [CrossRef] [PubMed]
16. Trussell, J.; Lalla, A.M.; Doan, Q.V.; Reyes, E.; Pinto, L.; Gricar, J. Cost effectiveness of contraceptives in the United States. *Contraception* **2009**, *79*, 5–14. [CrossRef] [PubMed]
17. Evans, M.L.; Espey, E.; Ogburn, T.; Zite, N.B. Use of Long-Acting Reversible Contraception by Obstetrics and Gynecology Residents: An Examination of Access for All Women. *Obstet. Gynecol.* **2018**, *131*, 538–541. [CrossRef] [PubMed]

18. Secura, G.M.; Allsworth, J.E.; Madden, T.; Mullersman, J.L.; Peipert, J.F. The Contraceptive CHOICE Project: Reducing barriers to long-acting reversible contraception. *Am. J. Obstet. Gynecol.* **2010**, *203*, 115.e1–115.e7. [CrossRef]
19. Peipert, J.F.; Zhao, Q.; Allsworth, J.E.; Petrosky, E.; Madden, T.; Eisenberg, D.; Secura, G. Continuation and satisfaction of reversible contraception. *Obstet. Gynecol.* **2011**, *117*, 1105–1113. [CrossRef] [PubMed]
20. Rosenstock, J.R.; Peipert, J.F.; Madden, T.; Zhao, Q.; Secura, G.M. Continuation of reversible contraception in teenagers and young women. *Obstet. Gynecol.* **2012**, *120*, 1298–1305. [CrossRef]
21. Curtis, K.M.; Tepper, N.K.; Jatlaoui, T.C.; Berry-Bibee, E.; Horton, L.G.; Zapata, L.B.; Simmons, K.B.; Pagano, H.P.; Jamieson, D.J.; Whiteman, M.K. US medical eligibility criteria for contraceptive use, 2016. *Morb. Mortal. Wkly. Rep. Recomm. Rep.* **2016**, *65*, 1–103. [CrossRef]
22. Lohr, P.A.; Lyus, R.; Prager, S. Use of intrauterine devices in nulliparous women. *Contraception* **2017**, *95*, 529–537. [CrossRef]
23. Logan, R.G.; Thompson, E.L.; Vamos, C.A.; Griner, S.B.; Vazquez-Otero, C.; Daley, E.M. Is Long-Acting Reversible Contraceptive Use Increasing? Assessing Trends Among U.S. College Women, 2008–2013. *Matern. Child Health J.* **2018**. [CrossRef] [PubMed]
24. Sonfield, A.; Kost, K.; Gold, R.B.; Finer, L.B. The Public Costs of Births Resulting from Unintended Pregnancies: National and State-Level Estimates. *Perspect. Sex. Reprod. Health* **2011**, *43*, 94–102. [CrossRef] [PubMed]
25. Dehlendorf, C.; Rodriguez, M.I.; Levy, K.; Borrero, S.; Steinauer, J. Disparities in family planning. *Am. J. Obstet. Gynecol.* **2010**, *202*, 214–220. [CrossRef] [PubMed]
26. Bergin, A.; Tristan, S.; Terplan, M.; Gilliam, M.L.; Whitaker, A.K. A missed opportunity for care: Two-visit IUD insertion protocols inhibit placement. *Contraception* **2012**, *86*, 694–697. [CrossRef] [PubMed]
27. Turok, D.K.; Eisenberg, D.L.; Teal, S.B.; Keder, L.M.; Creinin, M.D. A prospective assessment of pelvic infection risk following same-day sexually transmitted infection testing and levonorgestrel intrauterine system placement. *Am. J. Obstet. Gynecol.* **2016**, *215*, 599.e1–599.e6. [CrossRef] [PubMed]
28. Jatlaoui, T.C.; Simmons, K.B.; Curtis, K.M. The safety of intrauterine contraception initiation among women with current asymptomatic cervical infections or at increased risk of sexually transmitted infections. *Contraception* **2016**, *94*, 701–712. [CrossRef]
29. American College of Obstetricians and Gynecologists. ACOG Practice Bulletin No. 121: Long-acting reversible contraception: Implants and intrauterine devices. *Obstet. Gynecol.* **2011**, *118*, 184–196. [CrossRef]
30. Romano, M.J.; Toye, P.; Patchen, L. Continuation of long-acting reversible contraceptives among Medicaid patients. *Contraception* **2018**. [CrossRef]
31. Hubacher, D. Copper intrauterine device use by nulliparous women: Review of side effects. *Contraception* **2007**, *75*, S8–S11. [CrossRef]
32. Hoggart, L.; Newton, V.L.; Dickson, J. "I think it depends on the body, with mine it didn't work": Explaining young women's contraceptive implant removal. *Contraception* **2013**, *88*, 636–640. [CrossRef]
33. Berenson, A.B.; Tan, A.; Hirth, J.M. Complications and continuation rates associated with 2 types of long-acting contraception. *Am. J. Obstet. Gynecol.* **2015**, *212*, 761.e1–761.e8. [CrossRef] [PubMed]
34. Chiles, D.P.; Roberts, T.A.; Klein, D.A. Initiation and continuation of long-acting reversible contraception in the United States military healthcare system. *Am. J. Obstet. Gynecol.* **2016**, *215*, 328.e1–328.e9. [CrossRef]
35. Grunloh, D.S.; Casner, T.; Secura, G.M.; Peipert, J.F.; Madden, T. Characteristics associated with discontinuation of long-acting reversible contraception within the first 6 months of use. *Obstet. Gynecol.* **2013**, *122*, 1214–1221. [CrossRef] [PubMed]
36. Amico, J.R.; Bennett, A.H.; Karasz, A.; Gold, M. "I wish they could hold on a little longer": physicians' experiences with requests for early IUD removal. *Contraception* **2017**, *96*, 106–110. [CrossRef] [PubMed]
37. Foster, D.G.; Grossman, D.; Turok, D.K.; Peipert, J.F.; Prine, L.; Schreiber, C.A.; Jackson, A.V.; Barar, R.E.; Schwarz, E.B. Interest in and experience with IUD self-removal. *Contraception* **2014**, *90*, 54–59. [CrossRef] [PubMed]
38. Curtis, K.M.; Jatlaoui, T.C.; Tepper, N.K.; Zapata, L.B.; Horton, L.G.; Jamieson, D.J.; Whiteman, M.K. U.S. Selected Practice Recommendations for Contraceptive Use, 2016. *Morb. Mortal. Wkly. Rep. Recomm. Rep.* **2016**, *65*, 1–66. [CrossRef]
39. Long-Acting Reversible Contraception Working Group. ACOG Committee Opinion no. 450: Increasing use of contraceptive implants and intrauterine devices to reduce unintended pregnancy. *Obstet. Gynecol.* **2009**, *114*, 1434–1438. [CrossRef] [PubMed]
40. Morroni, C.; Findley, M.; Westhoff, C. Does using the "pregnancy checklist" delay safe initiation of contraception? *Contraception* **2017**, *95*, 331–334. [CrossRef] [PubMed]
41. Amico, J.; Wu, J. Providing Long-Acting Reversible Contraception in an Academic Family Medicine Center. *Fam. Med.* **2015**, *47*, 727–731.
42. Raine, T.R.; Foster-Rosales, A.; Upadhyay, U.D.; Boyer, C.B.; Brown, B.A.; Sokoloff, A.; Harper, C.C. One-year contraceptive continuation and pregnancy in adolescent girls and women initiating hormonal contraceptives. *Obstet. Gynecol.* **2011**, *117*, 363–371. [CrossRef]
43. American College of Obstetricians and Gynecologists. Committee opinion no. 539: Adolescents and long-acting reversible contraception: Implants and intrauterine devices. *Obstet. Gynecol.* **2012**, *120*, 983–988. [CrossRef] [PubMed]
44. Dickerson, L.M.; Diaz, V.A.; Jordon, J.; Davis, E.; Chirina, S.; Goddard, J.A.; Carr, K.B.; Carek, P.J. Satisfaction, early removal, and side effects associated with long-acting reversible contraception. *Fam. Med.* **2013**, *45*, 701–707. [PubMed]
45. Peterson, H.B.; Cates, W. Evidence-based medicine in action: The United States Selected Practice Recommendations for Contraceptive Use. *Contraception* **2013**, *87*, 509–510. [CrossRef] [PubMed]

46. Battaglia, C.; Battaglia, B.; Casadio, P.; Rizzo, R.; Artini, P.G. Metformin metabolic and vascular effects in normal weight hyperinsulinemic polycystic ovary syndrome patients treated with contraceptive vaginal ring. A pilot study. *Gynecol. Endocrinol.* **2020**, *36*, 1062–1069. [CrossRef]
47. Morotti, E.; Casadio, P.; Guasina, F.; Battaglia, B.; Mattioli, M.; Battaglia, C. Weight gain, body image and sexual function in young patients treated with contraceptive vaginal ring. A prospective pilot study. *Gynecol. Endocrinol.* **2017**, *33*, 660–664. [CrossRef]
48. Battaglia, C.; Morotti, E.; Persico, N.; Battaglia, B.; Busacchi, P.; Casadio, P.; Paradisi, R.; Venturoli, S. Clitoral vascularization and sexual behavior in young patients treated with drospirenone-ethinyl estradiol or contraceptive vaginal ring: A prospective, randomized, pilot study. *J. Sex. Med.* **2014**, *11*, 471–480. [CrossRef]
49. Amico, J.R.; Bennett, A.H.; Karasz, A.; Gold, M. Taking the provider "out of the loop:" patients' and physicians' perspectives about IUD self-removal. *Contraception* **2018**. [CrossRef]
50. Godfrey, E.M.; West, I.I.; Holmes, J.; Keppel, G.A.; Baldwin, L.M. Use of an electronic health record data sharing system for identifying current contraceptive use within the WWAMI region Practice and Research Network. *Contraception* **2018**, *98*, 476–481. [CrossRef]

Article

Utility of the Levonorgestrel-Releasing Intrauterine System in the Treatment of Abnormal Uterine Bleeding and Dysmenorrhea: A Narrative Review

Paola Bianchi [1,*], Sun-Wei Guo [2,3], Marwan Habiba [4] and Giuseppe Benagiano [5]

1. Department of Medico-Surgical Sciences and Translational Medicine, Sant'Andrea Hospital, Sapienza, University of Rome, 00161 Rome, Italy
2. Shanghai OB/GYN Hospital, Fudan University, Shanghai 200011, China
3. Shanghai Key Laboratory of Female Reproductive Endocrine-Related Diseases, Fudan University, Shanghai 200011, China
4. Department of Health Sciences, University Hospitals of Leicester, University of Leicester, Leicester LE1 7RH, UK
5. Faculty of Medicine and Dentistry, Sapienza, University of Rome, 00161 Rome, Italy
* Correspondence: paola.bianchi@uniroma1.it

Abstract: Introduction: We undertook a literature review of the use of levonorgestrel-releasing intrauterine devices when utilized for heavy menstrual bleeding and/or dysmenorrhea. Methods: A narrative review of articles in the Scopus and Medline databases was conducted. Results: A number of options exist for the management of both abnormal uterine bleeding (AUB) and dysmenorrhea, and evidence is accumulating that the insertion of a levonorgestrel-releasing intrauterine system (LNG-IUS) represents a useful option for their long-term treatment. The idea of using a progestogen released in utero was initially conceived to achieve long-term contraception, but it was quickly found that these systems could be utilized for a number of therapeutic applications. The first device to be made commercially available, Progestasert, was withdrawn from the market because, in the event of contraceptive failure, it caused a disproportionate percentage of extrauterine pregnancies. On the other hand, the LNG-IUS continues to be successfully utilized in its various variants, releasing 20, 13, or 8 µg/day. These devices have a respective duration of action of 7 (possibly 8), 5, and 3 years, and there exist versions of frameless systems affixed to the myometrium of the uterine fundus. In the present review, following a brief description of the major causes of AUB and dysmenorrhea, the molecular bases for the use of the LNG-IUS are summarized. This is followed by a compendium of its use in AUB and dysmenorrhea, concluding that the insertion of the system improves the quality of life, reduces menstrual blood loss better than other medical therapies, and decreases the extent of dysmenorrhea and pelvic pain. In addition, there is no evidence of a significant difference in these outcomes when the use of the LNG-IUS was compared with improvements offered by endometrial ablation or hysterectomy. Possibly, the most important mechanism of action of the system consists of its ability to induce amenorrhea, which effectively eliminates heavy bleeding and dysmenorrhea. However, no method is ideal for every woman, and, in the case of the LNG-IUS, younger age and severe dysmenorrhea seem to be associated with a higher risk of discontinuation. Conclusion: The higher-dose LNG-IUS is a useful tool for HMB and dysmenorrhea in women of all ages. The low cost and ease of use make the LNG-IUS an attractive option, especially when contraception is also desired.

Keywords: abnormal uterine bleeding; amenorrhea; dysmenorrhea; levonorgestrel-releasing intrauterine system; Progestasert

1. Introduction

In their recent comprehensive review of the regulation of menstruation, Critchley et al. [1] reminded us that the menstruating endometrium is a physiological example of an injured or "wounded" surface requiring rapid repair each month. They also pointed out that abnormal uterine bleeding (AUB) imposes a massive burden on one in four women of reproductive age. The estimates by Davis and Sparzaks [2] indicate that up to 1/3 of all women will experience some form of AUB in their lifetime, most commonly around menarche and perimenopause.

In addition, a comprehensive review of longitudinal, case–control, and cross-sectional studies found a wide difference of between 16% and 91% in the prevalence of dysmenorrhea in women of reproductive age and that 2–29% of them suffered severe pain. Factors linked to reduced risk are older age, higher parity, and the use of oral contraceptives. High stress and a family history increase the risk of dysmenorrhea. There is inconclusive evidence about the role of smoking, diet, obesity, depression, or abuse [3]. Dysmenorrhea affects women across the globe [3,4].

In recognition of the magnitude of the problem, the plethora of possible and often coexisting causes and the inconsistency in the nomenclature used to describe AUB, the International Federation of Gynecologists and Obstetricians (FIGO) [5] proposed a comprehensive classification system aimed at facilitating both clinical care and research coined the "PALM-COEIN" (polyp; adenomyosis; leiomyoma; malignancy and hyperplasia; coagulopathy; ovulatory dysfunction; endometrial; iatrogenic; and not yet classified). It systematically classifies AUB into groups with distinctively different structural and functional causes. Recently, FIGO also proposed a new classification for ovulatory disorders [6].

An illustration of the PALM-COEIN system is provided in Figure 1.

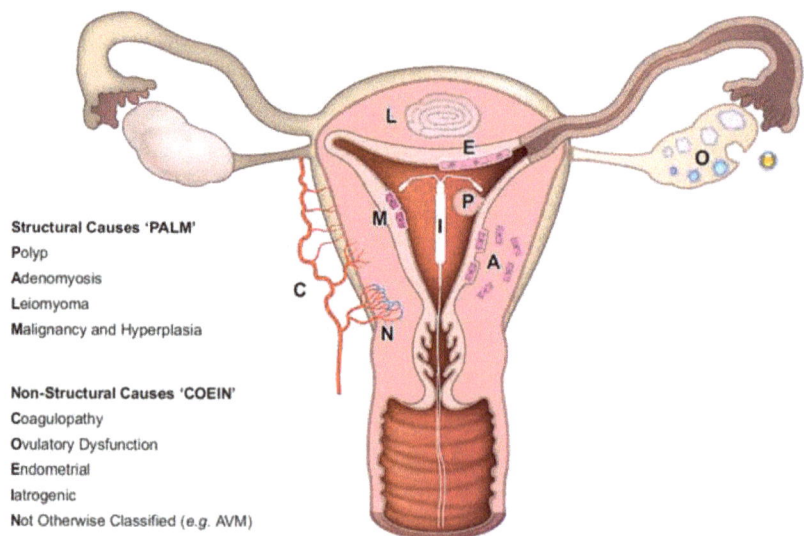

Figure 1. Illustration of the PALM-COEN classification system for abnormal uterine bleeding. From Critchley et al. (2020) [1] (reproduced with permission).

A number of options exist for the management of both AUB and dysmenorrhea. In 2016, Bradley and Gueye [7] summarized the process of dealing with the two conditions as follows: Take a thorough history and perform a physical examination and proper imaging studies; once all significant structural causes are excluded, proceed with medical management. In the presence of an acute episode of AUB with a normal uterus, parenteral estrogen, multidose combined oral contraceptives (COCs), multidose progestin-only regimen, and tranexamic acid are all indicated. If heavy bleeding is a common feature, then a levonorgestrel-releasing intrauterine system (LNG-IUS), COCs, continuous oral progestins, and tranexamic acid represent efficacious methods.

With regard to dysmenorrhea, a recent review by McKenna and Fogleman [8] recommended starting with the menstrual history and a pregnancy test for sexually active patients, followed by nonsteroidal anti-inflammatory drugs (NSAIDs), COCs, and an LNG-IUS, all considered first-line medical options.

In clinical practice, AUB and dysmenorrhea often coexist [9], and therefore, from a practical point of view, the same treatment can be applied in the presence of both symptoms. It should be noted that both conditions represent important non-contraceptive indications of pharmacological agents that were first utilized for fertility regulation. Such applications have been known for decades and were systematically listed in 2010 by the American College of Obstetricians and Gynecologists (ACOG), which provided a comprehensive list of such benefits [10,11]. Specifically, they affirmed that *"Hormonal contraception should be considered for women with menorrhagia who may desire future pregnancies . . . Data on the effects of the levonorgestrel intrauterine system on dysmenorrhea are limited, but because the device reduces or eliminates menstruation for many women, these benefits seem consistent with the mechanism of action . . . The levonorgestrel intrauterine system reduces blood loss by up to 86 percent after three months, and by up to 97 percent after 12 months"*.

In the last few years, new drugs, such as dienogest, selective progesterone receptor modulators (SPRMs), and GnRH antagonists, have become available for the management of HMB and dysmenorrhea due to uterine fibroids and adenomyosis. However, the use of SPRMs is restricted by European Medicine Agency (EMA) warnings, and GnRH antagonists are still very pricy. Given the importance of the benefits of the LNG-IUS for these two indications and its low cost and excellent safety profile, we decided to critically review the molecular, biological, and clinical information on the use of the LNG-IUS to treat AUB and dysmenorrhea.

2. Methods

This narrative review is based on articles identified through a search of Scopus and Medline databases until March 2022 using the headings HMB, menorrhagia, dysmenorrhea, and AUB, together with levonorgestrel (or norgestrel) intrauterine device or system and progestogen intrauterine device or system. We searched for major publications, including systematic reviews, meta-analyses, randomized controlled trials (RCTs), and consensus concerning the utility of the LNG-IUS in the treatment of abnormal uterine bleeding and dysmenorrhea. The reference lists of identified articles were used to search for any additional relevant references. Articles published in languages other than English were excluded. This article consists of a narrative review to synthesize the findings in the literature, which was conducted following the Scale for Assessment of Narrative Review Articles (SANRA).

3. Definition and Management of Abnormal Uterine Bleeding

As mentioned, there is a comprehensive definition and classification system for all types of AUB, "PALM-COEIN" [5]. More specifically, Warner et al. [12,13] defined the most common form, menorrhagia (a term increasingly replaced by the expression: "heavy menstrual bleeding", HMB), in terms of a statistical "abnormality", namely, as a blood loss of >80 mL per cycle, as first investigated by Hallberg et al. more than 50 years ago [14]. The use of the term "menorrhagia" should be discouraged, as it has been applied loosely, notwithstanding the fact that it does have a precise definition.

In routine clinical practice, measurements are seldom carried out. Warner et al. [12] found that, in their cohort, only 34% (95% Confidence Interval (CI) = 28–40%) of women had a volume of blood loss >80 mL, associated with the subjective heaviness of the period. Women reported a range of problems associated with their periods [14]: dysmenorrhea (37.5%), mood changes (35.7%), and changes over time in the amount (volume) of menses

(33.8%). Interestingly, the absolute volume was only fourth among their complaints (31.2%). They concluded that the 80 mL criterion for menorrhagia is of limited clinical usefulness, since it does not predict the presence of problems or the iron status. Therefore, it does not help in guiding management [13].

In contemporary times, HMB has been defined as excessive menstrual blood loss (MBL) that disrupts the physical, social, emotional, and/or material quality of life [15]. Over the years, a number of guidelines have been produced to manage HMB (e.g., [15–17]), and excellent reviews on the subject have been published [18–22].

Of particular relevance here is the Cochrane review of the use of progestogen-releasing intrauterine systems by Bofill Rodriguez et al. [23] that included 25 randomized clinical trials (RCTs), totaling 2511 women, comparing the LNG-IUS versus other medical therapies. They concluded that the LNG-IUS may improve HMB, lowering the MBL measured through the alkaline hematin method (mean difference (MD) 66.91 mL; 95% CI = 42.61–91.20) and the Pictorial Bleeding Assessment Chart (PBAC) (mean = 55.05; 95% CI = 27.83–82.28). The use of the LNG-IUS may have a favorable effect on women's satisfaction for up to one year (RR = 1.28; 95% CI = 1.01–1.63) and result in a slightly higher quality of life.

The definition of heavy menstrual bleeding has evolved over time. The current interpretation places it within the broad classification of abnormal uterine bleeding or AUB.

4. Definition and Management of Dysmenorrhea

Dysmenorrhea is defined by the presence of pain during menstruation. Pain can start before the onset of bleeding. It represents the most common menstrual symptom among adolescent girls and young women. If painful menstruation occurs in the absence of pelvic pathology, this is referred to as primary dysmenorrhea [24,25]. Dysmenorrhea is a common, often debilitating condition affecting between 45 and 95% of menstruating women, and it is often poorly treated or even disregarded in spite of its impact [24].

Following a critical review of published information, Iacovides et al. [24] concluded that women with primary dysmenorrhea acquire a greater sensitivity to pain both within and outside the period of menstruation. This leads to a significantly reduced quality of life, poorer mood, and poorer sleep quality during menstruation. In their view, the first-line treatment consists of the use of NSAIDs.

Guidelines for the management of dysmenorrhea have been produced by the UK National Institute for Health and Care Excellence (NICE) [25]; in addition, ACOG issued an opinion on how to manage dysmenorrhea associated with endometriosis in adolescent girls [26].

The management of endometriosis-associated pelvic pain and dysmenorrhea has been specifically investigated by Bahamondes and his group [27–29]. First, they investigated the use of biomarkers by measuring the serum levels of cancer antigen-125 (CA-125), cluster of differentiation 23 (CD23), and the endometrial nerve fiber (ENF) density before and after the insertion of the LNG-IUS or the etonogestrel (ENG) contraceptive implant. They observed that both systems significantly reduced the concentration of serum-soluble CD23 and the ENF density ($p < 0.001$); interestingly, CA-125 was significantly reduced only among users of the ENG implant ($p < 0.05$). Unfortunately, no correlation was observed between the reduction in biomarkers and improvements in visual analog scale (VAS) pain and dysmenorrhea scores. They then carried out a randomized comparative clinical trial of the ENG implant and the LNG-IUS and found that both systems significantly improved the mean VAS score. In addition, health-related quality of life improved significantly, with the most common bleeding pattern for the LNG-IUS at 180 days of follow-up being infrequent bleeding and spotting, as shown in Figure 2.

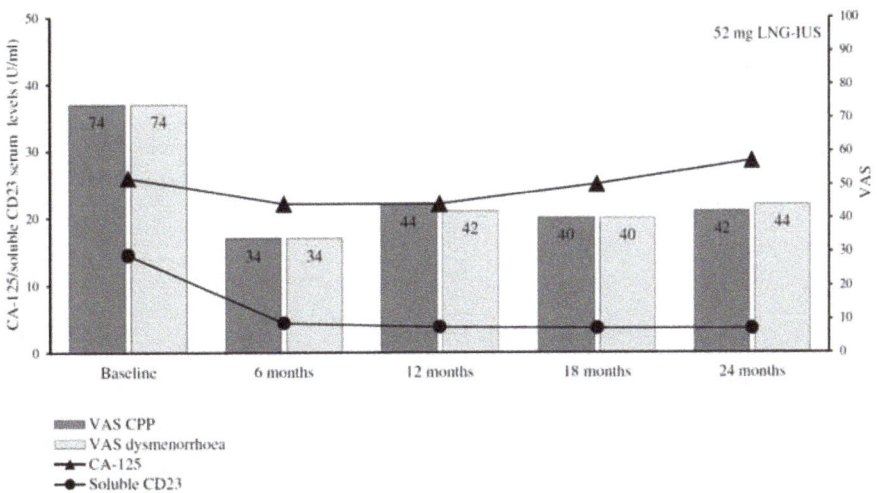

Figure 2. Serum levels of cancer antigen-125 (CA-125), cluster of differentiation 23 (CD23), visual analog scale (VAS), and chronic pelvic pain (CPP) over two years of treatment with the LNG-IUS. From: Margatho et al. (2020) [28] (reproduced with permission).

Dysmenorrhea is a very common presentation and is linked to a reduced quality of life. The use of the LNG-IUS improves the quality of life and pain scores, but there is no correlation with pain biomarkers.

5. The Progesterone-Releasing Intrauterine System

Contrary to a commonly held view, the concept of using a progestogen released in utero for contraception dates back more than fifty years: the first experimental device, reported in 1968, utilized medroxyprogesterone acetate (MPA) [30], but the initial system was abandoned because all of the devices were expelled within a month [31]. More successful were the attempts to first use a Lippes loop and then use the so-called Tatum-T as carriers for progesterone [32,33]. A progesterone-releasing device called Progestasert was marketed in the mid-1980s by Alza Corporation with a stated duration of one year [34]. It had a 1.3% failure rate, but quickly became the therapeutic device of choice for women with dysmenorrhea or heavy menstrual flow [35]. Unfortunately, epidemiological data evidenced that, in the event of contraceptive failure, the device caused a disproportionate percentage of extrauterine pregnancies [36], and, not withstanding its secondary therapeutic action, it was withdrawn from the market.

In spite of its short commercial life, a number of interesting observations of the biological effects of Progestasert were published. In particular, the mechanism of action was evaluated in the 1970s and 1980s, showing that, with time, the intrauterine administration of progesterone causes the increasing suppression of the proliferative activity of the endometrium, a clear pre-decidual stromal reaction, poorly developed glands, and a decrease in vascularity, accompanied by an increase in the proportion of small vessels with defects [37–40]. However, in a controlled study, the overall concentration of these small blood vessels was significantly lower than in normal subjects, with an average blood vessel density of 2.39 (range, 13.0 to 3.71) compared to 3.92 for the controls (range, 3.33 to 4.68) ($p = 0.01$) [40]. This led the authors to suggest that this phenomenon may account for significantly less uterine blood loss in Progestasert users. The proportion of defective vessels in controls ranged between 0% and 24%, and in the Progestasert group varied from 7.1% to 64%, with average percentages of 13.4% and 35.0%, respectively ($p = 0.001$).

In conclusion, the early stages of development of progestogen-releasing devices utilized MPA; this was followed by the use of progesterone microcrystals. The development of both types of devices was discontinued because of high expulsion rates in the case of the MPA device and because of the increased risk of ectopic pregnancy with the progesterone device.

6. Levonorgestrel-Releasing Intrauterine Systems

In 1975, an international group under the auspices of the Population Council [41] began testing a polylactate film releasing levonorgestrel (LNG) (in those days, called D-norgestrel), with the rates of the diffusion of the steroid and of the hydrolysis of the polymer suggesting that it could be utilized for intrauterine contraception. As a carrier, they used a copper-releasing T device stripped of the copper wire. The initial work showed promise for developing an intrauterine device capable of slowly releasing LNG over a period of 2–3 years.

In the following year, the same group [42] carried out a Phase I clinical trial in six women volunteers using a device composed of a Tatum-T-IUD in which the carrier for LNG was a sleeve of poly-dimethyl-siloxane (Silastic). The device was tested in six healthy women, and plasma concentrations of d-norgestrel (today renamed levonorgestrel), estradiol, and progesterone were determined for periods of 112–114 days. They observed plasma values of the steroid corresponding to a daily release of 50 pg, sufficient to suppress ovulation and produce irregular but reduced bleeding.

Since the early experience, it has become clear that the system has a positive effect on the amount of blood loss, as documented by Nilsson [43] (See Figure 3).

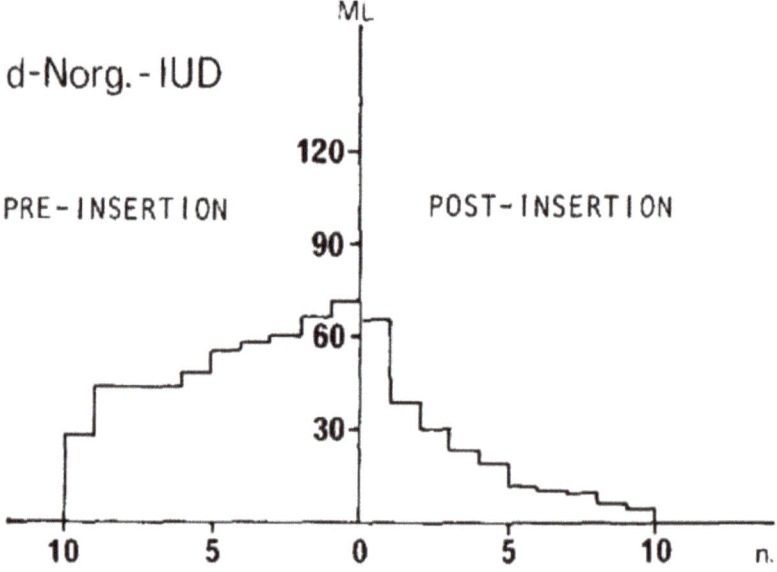

Figure 3. Duration and intensity of menstrual blood loss before and during 3 cycles after insertion of an experimental levonorgestrel-releasing device. From: Nilsson (1977) [42] (reproduced with permission).

Endometrial changes were also evaluated with devices releasing either 20 or 40 µg/day, observing a uniform suppression of the endometrium with glandular atrophy and the decidualization of the stroma [44].

By 1986, information had become available proving that the device's effectiveness as a contraceptive lasted 5 years [45], and in 2021, the US Food and Drug Administration

(FDA) approved its use for contraception for up 8 years [46,47] following the publication of evidence of its long-term effectiveness [48]. When used for HMB, the license is for 5 years.

As mentioned, a reduction in MBL has been observed since the very early clinical experience, and this led to the utilization of the device in subjects with HMB. The first application dealt with the prevention and treatment of iron-deficiency anemia [49], followed by the publication of the results of the use of the LNG-IUS for 1 year in a small cohort of 20 women with menorrhagia (>80 mL blood loss per menstrual period). There was a significant reduction in blood loss, reaching 97% at 1 year, when, in addition, there was also a significant increase ($p < 0.001$) in serum ferritin [50]. Soon afterward, it was proven that the reduction in MBL achieved by the LNG-IUS was significantly greater than that recorded with flurbiprofen ($p < 0.001$) and tranexamic acid ($p < 0.01$) [51].

By the turn of the millennium, besides menorrhagia and iron-deficiency anemia, several additional therapeutic indications were identified; these included: protection of the endometrium in estrogen replacement therapy; dysmenorrhea; endometrial hyperplasia; ovarian endometrioma; adenomyosis; and endometrial protection in women treated with tamoxifen during breast cancer treatment [52,53]. In a comprehensive review published in 2006 [54], additional indications were mentioned: fibroid-related menorrhagia, pelvic-inflammatory disease (not proven), and endometrial cancer. A number of reviews confirmed these indications [55–59]. However, caution should be exercised in women with malignancy, and whilst it may reduce endometriosis-related pain, it does not resolve endometriomas.

An interesting point was raised by Cristobal et al. [60], who prospectively evaluated the quality of life (QoL) of LNG-IUS users over the first-year post-insertion using the so-called "Spanish society of contraception quality-of-life" questionnaire, developed to specifically assess the impact of contraceptive methods on the health-related (HR) QoL. This index rose from a mean of 46.3 (±17.3) at baseline to 72.2 (±14.8) at 12 months ($p < 0.001$). Overall, 94.6% of the participating women claimed to have received additional benefits besides contraception.

In conclusion, as stressed by Gemzell-Danielsson et al. [61], the availability of the LNG-IUS has had a considerable impact on women's wellbeing far beyond the reduction in the need for abortion and surgical sterilization. It reduced the number of hysterectomies carried out for HMB and, in the context of the COVID-19 pandemic, provided a treatment option for women with some gynecological issues without organic pathology, minimizing their exposure to the hospital environment and waiting times for surgical appointments.

The successful development of the LNG-IUS has had a considerable impact beyond its use as an effective contraceptive. The LNG-IUS has proven to be an effective alternative to hysterectomy for HMB.

Type of Devices Available

The characteristics of levonorgestrel-releasing intrauterine systems (LNG-IUSs) available at present are summarized in Table 1.

Basically, four types of systems have been marketed: the first three utilize a T-shaped IUD, the vertical arm of which contains different quantities of LNG:

(1) **LNG-IUS-20**: Total content of 52.5 mg; LNG is initially released at a rate of 20 µg/day, and—as already mentioned—in 2021, the US FDA approved its use for contraception for up to 8 years [47]. It is licensed for HMB for up to 5 years.
(2) **LNG-IUS 12**: Total content of 19.5 mg; LNG is initially released at a rate of 13 µg/day and has a duration of action of 5 years [62]. The device is not licensed for HMB.
(3) **LNG-IUS 8**: Total content of 13.5 mg; LNG is initially released at a rate of 8 µg/day and has a duration of action of 3 years [63]. The device is not licensed for HMB.

Table 1. Various types of devices available on the market.

LNG-IUS 20: Total content: 52.5 mg; daily LNG release: 20 µg; FDA-approved duration of use: 8 years for contraception, 5 years for HMB. Available as: • *Mirena*® (Bayer, Germany); • *Levosert*® (Gedeon Richter) (known as *Donasert*® in Russia and France; *Benilexa*® in Italy; and *Liletta*® in the United States).
LNG-IUS 12: Total content: 19.5 mg; daily LNG release: 13µg; duration of use: 5 years (for contraception). Available as: • *Kayleena*® (Bayer).
LNG-IUS 8: Total content: 13.5 mg; daily LNG release: 8µg; duration of use: 3 years (for contraception). Available as: • *Jaydess*®*(Bayer)*; • *Skyla*®*(Bayer)*.
Frameless 3.5 cm-long coaxial fibrous LNG-IUS: Daily LNG release: 14µg; duration of use: 3 years. Available as: • *Fibroplant*®*(Contrel Research)*; • *GyneFix (Tianjin Medic, Medical Equipment Co., Ltd.)*.

The fourth system consists of a 3.5 cm-long coaxial fibrous LNG delivery system with an approximate release of 14 µg/day. The calculated duration of release from the device is at least 3 years [64].

In China, a similar frameless LNG-IUS affixed to the myometrium has been tested in patients with adenomyosis and HMB [65] in a comparative trial of 60-month duration. They observed, at 1-year, significant changes in the pretreatment severity of dysmenorrhea, menstrual volume, uterine volume, and hemoglobin level in each group ($p < 0.01$ in all groups).

The introduction of frameless devices is claimed to overcome cramps as a symptom in some users of framed devices. It may also be suitable in the presence of fibroids that distort the uterine cavity [66].

As shown in Table 1, the original LNG-IUS, commercially known as Mirena©, is currently marketed along with generic versions. Ilyin et al. [67] compared these generic systems with the reference product Mirena© in subjects with HMB. They randomly assigned Donasert or Mirena to a total of 312 subjects and observed mean absolute changes in MBL of −130 (71.8) mL and −127 (67.3) mL at 6 months in the Donasert and Mirena groups, respectively; the non-inferiority of Donasert was confirmed (p-value < 0.0001).

Recently, the WHO recommended that the classification system used for intrauterine contraception be made clearer. For instance, the WHO recommended that the type of hormone be specified (e.g., levonorgestrel-releasing IUD) [68]. The recommendation of the Society of Family Planning in the USA recommended that the dose release also be specified and that the word "releasing" be dropped. Thus, available devices would be referred to as Levonorgestrel 13.5 mg, 19.5 mg, or 52 mg IUDs [69]. It is important here to reiterate that the release rate constantly decreases with the duration of hormonal IUD use.

7. Causes of HMB and Dysmenorrhea and the Molecular Basis for the Use of LNG-IUS

As seen from the FIGO classification, the causes of AUB can be attributable to PALM-COEIN [70]. HMB is probably the most common form of AUB. The FIGO classification system lists the contributing causes of AUB (except for those instances that are not yet classified), but the underlying mechanisms are incompletely understood.

HMB has been linked to systemic causes, including hematological or thyroid disorders, as well as local uterine causes, such as fibroids or adenomyosis. However, a large proportion of women with HMB have no systemic or structural abnormalities, and the underlying mechanisms reside in the endometrium.

Following progesterone withdrawal in the late secretory phase in the absence of pregnancy, the endometrial expression of cyclooxygenase-2 (COX-2), a gene coding for the rate-limiting prostanoid-synthesizing enzyme, is elevated, resulting in subsequent increased levels of prostaglandins (PGs), particularly PGE_2 and $PGF_{2\alpha}$ [71,72]. The induction of endometrial PGE_2 signaling, along with the endometrial generation of the vasoconstrictor $PGF_{2\alpha}$, leads to local hypoxia in the upper functional layer of the endometrium. This is marked by the activation of hypoxia-inducible factor 1α (HIF-1α), the master regulator of cellular hypoxia, which, as such, establishes an endometrial microenvironment that is conducive to tissue repair and angiogenesis [73,74]. However, any disruption of hypoxia signaling or PGE_2 signaling in the endometrium will impair endometrial repair, causing HMB [1,75].

However, despite this knowledge, the more detailed mechanisms underlying adenomyosis-, endometrial-polyp-, and uterine-fibroid-induced HMB are largely unknown. For example, submucosal fibroids are more likely to be associated with HMB [76], but why this is so is less clear. However, a recent study indicates that the increased lesional fibrosis in adenomyosis, especially when located near the endometrium, can disrupt hypoxia and PGE_2 signaling, causing HMB [77]. This is because increased lesional fibrosis creates a microenvironment conducive to further fibrogenesis in neighboring tissues and a stiffened extracellular matrix (ECM), which, in turn, accentuates the actions of transforming growth factor β1 (TGF-β1) and promotes myofibroblast activation [78–80]. As a result, lesional fibrosis will propagate to the neighboring endometrial–myometrial interface (EMI) and then to the eutopic endometrium. As the matrix stiffness increases and interferes with multiple steps of PGE_2 synthesis, including the suppression of prostaglandin E synthases (PTGESs) that specifically convert the precursor PGH_2 to PGE_2 [81], PGE_2 production and signaling subside [82–85]. Increased fibrosis may also enhance PGE_2 degradation, as seen in the increased expression of the PGE_2-degrading enzyme 15-hydroxy-prostaglandin dehydrogenase (PGDH) in the fibrotic lung [85]. As a result, there will be a subsequent suppression of PGE_2,s as well as HIF-1α signaling in adenomyotic lesions and their EMI and endometrium, with ensuing impaired endometrial repair and, ultimately, HMB. Indeed, endometriotic stromal cells cultured on a stiff matrix display reduced expression of COX-2, prostaglandin E2 receptor 2 (EP2), and EP4 [83]. It is suspected that a similar mechanism may also be at work for submucosal fibroids [77].

The molecular mechanisms underlying dysmenorrhea are thought to be more complex. Conceivably, however, uterine hyperactivity, hyperinnervation within the uterus, the release of inflammatory cytokines and pain mediators by fibroids or adenomyotic lesions, and central sensitization may collectively contribute to dysmenorrhea.

The high local concentration of the progestin steadily released by the LNG-IUS suppresses the cellular proliferation of endometrial cells [86], thus inhibiting endometrial growth and resulting in a thinner endometrium. In addition, the pseudo-pregnancy (leading to pseudo-decidualization) conferred by the LNG-IUS results in no endometrial injury and thus no or substantially less bleeding. Moreover, the progestin released by the LNG-IUS changes the prostaglandin ratio by stimulating arachidonic acid formation in the endometrium [87] in favor of endometrial repair and thus less MBL.

The progestins contained in the LNG-IUS can also suppress uterine contractility [88–90], removing one important irritant that contributes to dysmenorrhea. Progestins can also activate progesterone receptors in the myometrium, antagonizing nuclear factor kappa-light-chain-enhancer of activated B cells (NF-κB) and thus reducing inflammation [91], removing another contributor to dysmenorrhea. As an added bonus for less or absent menstrual bleeding, there is less platelet aggregation and reduced or attenuated thrombin activation, which may further hinder uterine contractions [92,93].

Progesterone is central in endometrial remodeling and acts on both the epithelial and stromal compartments. Since a progestin is the major active agent within LNG-IUS, and since the action of progesterone/progestins is mediated through progesterone receptors (PRs), the ultimate efficacy of the LNG-IUS hinges critically on the expression levels of PRs, particularly PR isoform B (PR-B) in the endometrium and myometrium. In both adenomyotic and endometriotic lesions [94,95] and in endometrial hyperplasia and endometrial cancer [96–98], as well as in endometrial polyps [99], PR expression is all reduced. Hence, the LNG-IUS-released progestin, as a ligand, is likely to induce PR expression and exerts its therapeutic effect.

However, in many cases, the induction of PR expression can be difficult, if not impossible. For example, PR-B has been reported to be hypermethylated [100,101] and presumably silenced in endometriotic and adenomyotic lesions. In adenomyotic lesions in particular, the response to progestin treatment hinges critically on the mutational status of Kras [102]. Since it is unlikely that the methylation status or the DNA sequence is changed by progestin treatment, progestins may not be effective in containing these lesions when genetic/epigenetic aberrations are present.

In addition, for uterine leiomyoma, progesterone/progestins may actually stimulate cellular proliferation and fibrogenesis, effectively accelerating the disease progression [103–105], although evidence is not univocal: On the one hand, high doses of the progestin MPA are capable of promoting leiomyoma growth [104]. On the other hand, there is evidence that long-term progestogen administration reduces the occurrence of fibroids [106–108], and MPA administration prevented any significant re-growth following the treatment of women with symptomatic fibroids with the short-acting Gn-RH super-agonist analog Buserelin [109]. Finally, it has been shown that an add-back therapy of progestins with GnRH agonists reverses the efficacy of GnRH agonists in reducing fibroid size [110,111]. That is, progesterone/progestins may actually facilitate the progression of uterine leiomyoma. Still, treatment can be effective in reducing HMB.

Then, why is the LNG-IUS still useful in treating HMB and dysmenorrhea caused by endometriosis, adenomyosis, or leiomyoma? The LNG-IUS is effective in reducing menstrual blood loss. Among women using the LNG-IUS for contraception, amenorrhea or spotting was reported in approximately 50% of users during the last 90 days of the first year after insertion; with time, 80% experienced amenorrhea, spotting, or light bleeding only [112]. After 60 months of follow-up, 96.2% of women with HMB experienced amenorrhea, oligomenorrhea, or spotting, whilst 95.8% and 93.3% of women with adenomyosis or fibroids reported improvements [113]. This may stop or reduce the release of inflammatory and pain mediators associated with menstruation and, as such, dysmenorrhea. As Brosens pointed out in 1997 [114], endometriosis is characterized by recurrent ectopic bleeding, and, as such, the suppression of recurrent menstrual bleeding is in itself efficient in the treatment of symptomatic endometriosis. For other causes of HMB or dysmenorrhea, the rationale remains true as well.

In conclusion, although the molecular mechanisms are incompletely understood, the LNG-IUS proved effective in primary and some cases of secondary dysmenorrhea and in reducing HMB, including in women with fibroids.

8. Use in Abnormal Uterine Bleeding

By the end of the previous millennium, several investigators had tested the use of the LNG-IUS in the treatment of AUB. In 1997, two reports provided evidence of a positive effect in subjects with heavy bleeding: Fedele et al. [115] inserted the device in 25 women with recurrent adenomyosis-related menorrhagia. Of the 23 women who completed 12 months of treatment, 2 had become amenorrheic, 3 were oligomenorrheic, 2 reported spotting, and 16 had regular periods. The authors speculated that the IUS produced decidualization and, subsequently, marked hypotrophy of the eutopic endometrium. Barrington and Bowen-Simpkins [116] inserted the LNG-IUS in 50 women awaiting surgery and evaluated menstrual loss using a pictorial chart, a full blood count, and the measurement of ferritin.

By nine months post-insertion, bleeding was reduced to acceptable levels in 41 cases, with 4 subjects developing amenorrhea. These results were subsequently confirmed in larger cohorts [117,118].

A series of investigations tested the efficacy of the LNG-IUS in women harboring leiomyomas, with interesting results [119–124]. With one exception [112], they all concluded that the insertion of the system was associated with a profound reduction in menstrual blood loss and a significant reduction in uterine volume. At the same time, the LNG-IUS does not significantly reduce the volume of leiomyomas. One investigation [124] found a significant reduction in visual bleeding scores and spotting with an increase in amenorrhea and uterine pulsatility index scores, whereas another [16] observed a drop in the PBAC from a mean value of 231.7 to 17.6 at 12 months. In addition, the duration of menstrual bleeding diminished significantly ($p < 0.001$), with a good satisfaction rate in 89% of all cases. It can be concluded that the LNG-IUS is effective in controlling both menorrhagia and/or frequent irregular uterine bleeding related to the presence of myomas, though with no significant effect on the myoma size.

In an RCT that included women with idiopathic HMB, the LNG-IUS was more effective than cyclical MPA given for 10 days starting from day 16 of the cycle. The LNG-IUS was linked to a greater absolute and percentage reduction in menstrual blood loss and a higher likelihood of success [125].

Using the "frameless" LNG-IUS, Wildemeersch and Schacht [126] evaluated a small group of 14 subjects with the device in place for more than 1 year and 29 subjects with the device for 6 months or more. All women reported greatly reduced blood loss, although there were no cases of amenorrhea; the reduction in bleeding was substantial after 1 month of treatment and further decreased over the next months to remain stable thereafter.

An interesting investigation aimed at determining whether the size of the uterine cavity is a determining factor in causing bleeding and pain in nulligravid women using the LNG-IUS [127], and the authors concluded that a small uterine cavity size is in fact beneficial, causing an increase in the rate of amenorrhea and decreasing the presence of pain. Recently, Beelen et al. [128], in a cohort of 201 women with HMB, observed a discontinuation rate of 46% at 24 months, with age <45 (adjusted RR = 1.51; 95% CI = 1.10–2.09; $p = 0.012$) and severe dysmenorrhea (adjusted RR = 1.36; 95% CI = 1.01–1.82; $p = 0.041$) being associated with a higher risk of discontinuation. Anticipatory counseling can reduce premature removal of the device.

A recent investigation enrolled a cohort of 1714 subjects and followed them for 5 years, with 495 participants finishing the entire period. As shown in Figure 4, the rate of amenorrhea among these women increased with time, and at the end of the five years, it almost reached 42% [129].

It is important to mention that Cho et al. [130], on the one hand, reported a significant reduction in pain scores, menstrual blood loss, and uterine volume in women with adenomyosis after one year of LNG-IUS insertion; on the other, they found a significant increase in all parameters at 36 months of use compared to 12 months, suggesting a reduction in efficacy in the longer term.

This may be due to a reduction over time in the amount of LNG released by the system. According to the FDA, the initial release of the steroid is 20 μg/day, but this is reduced to around 10 ug/day over time. In terms of plasma levels, from the initial 150–200 pg/mL during the first weeks, there is a reduction to 180 ± 66 pg/mL, 192 ± 140 pg/mL, and 159 ± 59 pg/mL at 12, 24, and 60 months, respectively [46].

To conclude, a 2015 systematic review [131] found that the use of the LNG-IUS improved the quality of life and reduced menstrual blood loss better than standard medical therapy. It also found no evidence of a significant difference in these outcomes when the use of the system was compared with the improvements offered by endometrial ablation or hysterectomy.

In conclusion, the effectiveness of the LNG-IUS in women with HMB is well documented, but anticipatory counseling is important for avoiding premature removal. The

LNG-IUS that releases 20 ug/day is required to control HMB. Its use is associated with endometrial pseudo-decidualization.

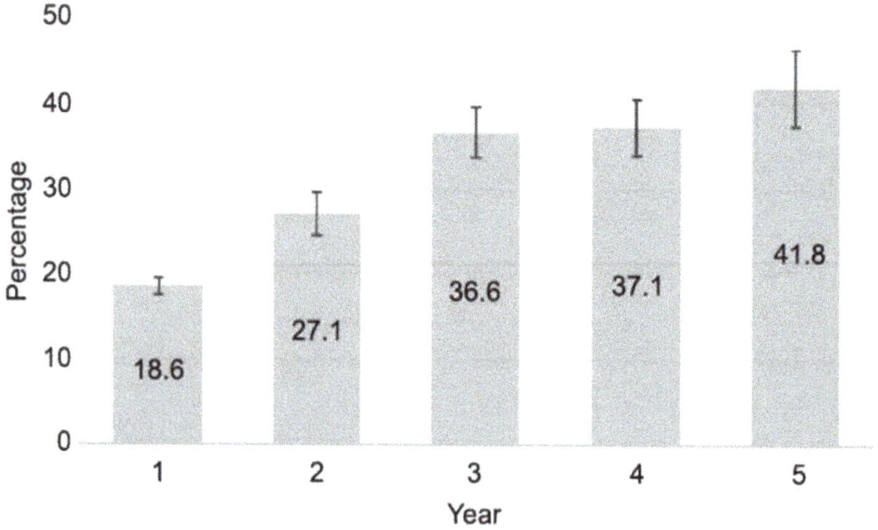

Figure 4. Rates of amenorrhea (defined as no bleeding or spotting during the preceding 90 days) over time in women bearing the LNG-IUS. From: Teal et al. (2019) [105] (reproduced with permission).

8.1. Use in Women with Bleeding Disorders

The link between abnormal bleeding and hematological disorders has been recognized for some time [132]. Attention to this phenomenon was drawn by a group of hematologists at the London Free Hospital around the turn of the millennium [133,134]. They reported that menorrhagia affected 74% of patients with von Willebrand disease (vWD), 57% of carriers of hemophilia A or B, 59% with Factor XI deficiency (FXID), and 60% with Factor VII deficiency, compared with 29% of control subjects.

At that time, tranexamic acid (TxA) and desmopressin acetate were utilized to control menorrhagia in these women; then, in 2004, the London Group, for the first time, proposed using the LNG-IUS [135]. They carried out a prospective pilot study in 16 women with treatment-resistant menorrhagia caused by the following inherited bleeding disorders (IBDs): vWD (n = 13), FXID (n = 2), and Hermansky–Pudlak syndrome, a genetic disorder characterized by, i.a., platelet dysfunction (n = 1). Subjects were followed up for nine months, and all women reported improvements in their periods, with lower pictorial chart scores; 56% became amenorrhoeic.

Soon after, another investigation explored the use of the LNG-IUS during anticoagulant therapy through the distribution of a questionnaire, with 17 responders [136]. The study reported that, following insertion, there was a reduction in bleeding in 10 women, and amenorrhea occurred in 4 cases. There was no change in one patient and an increase in bleeding in the last two. By 2007, Kadir and Chi [137] had identified four studies suggesting that the LNG-IUS is a viable and safe option for the management of menorrhagia in women with IBDs. Additional cases were published by Lukes et al. [138].

The results of the long-term follow-up (mean duration of 33 months; range: 14–103) of 26 subjects with IBDs were presented by Chi et al. [139]: they found that while using the LNG-IUS, the median PBAC score decreased from 255 (range, 134–683) to 35 (range, 0–89); the median hemoglobin (Hb) concentrations rose from 11.2 to 13.2 g/dL, and the QoL scores improved significantly, with the median rising from 26 to 52 ($p < 0.01$).

Two important complications of the LNG-IUS in these subjects, malposition and expulsion, were evaluated by Rimmer et al. [140], starting from the accepted expulsion rates of between 5 and 10% in normal subjects. The majority of subjects studied (12/20) were affected by type 1 VWD; their median age at the time of insertion was 31 years (range 18–43 years). There were three LNG-IUS expulsions and two episodes of device malposition resulting in removal (25.0%). An additional five women had their devices removed prematurely. From this study, it seems that a significant proportion of women with an IBD had the device removed due to malposition or expulsion. Obviously, the small number of subjects (a common feature of all investigations in IBD women) suggests caution in assessing these figures.

A small study from China reported on the successful use of the LNG-IUS in two adolescents with Glanzmann's Thrombasthenia, an IBD caused by defects in the platelet membrane glycoproteins IIb/IIIA. Insertion of the system produced a significant reduction in menstrual blood loss [141]. Another Chinese report [142] mentioned the case of a woman affected by primary myelofibrosis, a rare condition secondary to progressive pancytopenia; she suffered from HMB in spite of using a COC, and the administration of norethisterone yielded an unsatisfactory hemostatic effect. At this stage, an LNG-IUS was inserted, and at the 5-month follow-up, the patient reported a lower menstruation bleeding volume.

With time, more substantial cohorts became available: Brull et al. [143] reviewed the charts of 117 women attending a clinic for reasons related to IBDs who used the LNG-IUS. Ninety-nine of them had a history of thrombosis (with 71.7% using oral anticoagulants), and eighteen had coagulopathies. Approximately two-thirds of these subjects reported amenorrhea or oligomenorrhea at 12, 24, and 54 months of follow-up. No difference was observed between the groups with a history of thrombosis or coagulopathy, or between users and non-users of oral anticoagulants. A second study [144] followed 20 subjects with IBDs wearing the LNG-IUS; they observed a progressive reduction in the median PBAC score over time, becoming highly significant at 12 months ($p < 0.001$). At that time, 70% of the subjects were amenorrheic. Finally, there was a substantial ($p < 0.001$) improvement in eight parameters of quality of life (QoL), as well as in the levels of hemoglobin, ferritin, and serum iron.

At present, guidelines are available for the gynecologic and obstetric management of women with vWD derived from three systematic reviews of the literature comparing the effects of desmopressin, hormonal therapy, and TxA on HMB [145]. When comparing desmopressin to COCs, a single observational study suggested that both are equally effective at alleviating symptoms (RR = 0.90; 95% CI = 0.66–1.23). With regard to the LNG-IUS, the review found that, unfortunately, case series could not be included in the meta-analysis. At any rate, they found very low certainty for the comparative effectiveness of the LNG-IUS with other therapies in the control of HMB, the duration of menstruation, health-related quality of life, anemia, absence from necessary activities, complications, and adverse effects.

8.2. The Effect of the LNG-IUS on the Endometrium

Locally released LNG has a profound effect on the endometrium: as already mentioned, back in 1978, changes in the endometrium were evaluated with devices releasing either 20 or 40 μg/day, observing a uniform suppression of the endometrium [44]. Under the influence of locally delivered LNG, there is a thinning of the mucosa to about 1–3 mm. The stroma becomes edematous and features pseudo-decidualization of the cells. The endometrial glands are scarce and atrophic with no mitosis, and there is leukocytic infiltration [146].

8.3. Comparison of Blood Loss with Cu-IUD

In an early investigation, Nilsson [43] quantified and compared menstrual blood loss with the LNG-IUS and a Nova-T-copper device (Cu-IUD) in a group of 19 volunteers and calculated, over three consecutive menstrual periods, a blood loss of 20.7 ± 6.0 mL for the former and 72.5 ± 6.2 mL for the latter. In addition, over time, the amount of blood loss significantly decreased during the use of the LNG-IUS.

Some 35 years later, Lowe and Prata [147] carried out a systematic review of changes in Hb and ferritin and compared the effects of the LNG-IUS with those of the Cu-IUD. They found 14 investigations involving the copper device in nonanemic subjects and 4 in anemic subjects; these were compared to the results of reviewing 6 trials of the levonorgestrel system. The meta-analyses for hemoglobin changes showed significant decreases for bearers of Cu-IUDs and an increase for the LNG-IUS. In the case of ferritin, the levels followed the same pattern. Interestingly, decreases in mean hemoglobin values in bearers of the copper device were not sufficient to induce anemia in previously nonanemic women.

An investigation in India [148] compared hemoglobin and ferritin in two groups of 50 subjects and found that the insertion of the LNG-IUS reduced the number of menstrual bleeding days and increased both hemoglobin and serum ferritin levels. Specifically, in users of the LNG-IUS, at one year, besides Hb and ferritin, there were also increases in red blood cells, packed cell volume, mean corpuscular volume, mean corpuscular hemoglobin, and mean corpuscular hemoglobin concentration, whereas the values of all of these parameters decreased in the Cu-IUD group. These observations may be especially important for women in developing countries, where a decrease in blood loss may improve iron-deficient conditions.

9. Use in Dysmenorrhea

The early investigation by Barrington and Bowen-Simpkins [116] observed that 56% of their cohort of 41 women noticed considerable improvements in, or the outright cure of their premenstrual syndrome symptoms, whereas 80% reported a reduction in the severity of dysmenorrhea (SDys). Ten years later, Bahamondes et al. [149] carried out a review of the medical literature on the effect of the LNG-IUS on pelvic pain and dysmenorrhea and found that all trials reported improvements in both parameters. One study with a follow-up of three years, while finding improvement in pelvic pain at 12 months of use, reported no further improvement after that.

Over the years, additional information has become available: Yucel et al. [150], in subjects with endometriomas, found a decrease in the VAS score of pain intensity from 6.13 to 2.88 and of dyspareunia from 6.04 to 2.61 at 12 months. Yoo et al. [151] focused their attention on the hysterectomy rates and the risk factors for hysterectomy during the first 2 years of use of the LNG-IUS in perimenopausal women complaining of either menorrhagia or dysmenorrhea. They found that out of 192 women over 40 years of age, 26 (13.5%) had to be hysterectomized because of the failure of the system; however, the severity of pain before treatment was not a factor for referral for surgery. On the other hand, surgery was correlated with the pain score at three months.

In a longitudinal population study, Lindh and Milsom [152] addressed a vital question: whether intrauterine contraception influences the prevalence of SDys. They compared SDys in the same woman using a Cu-IUD, the LNG-IUS, or a COC with other methods of contraception or no contraception. Intriguingly, they found that SDys was unchanged in the same women when using a Cu-IUD compared with using other methods (condom, barrier methods, natural family planning, coitus interruptus, and sterilization) or no method of contraception. LNG-IUS and COC use were associated with reduced SDys compared with other methods/no method. Finally, SDys decreased between the ages of 19 and 44 years.

Kelekci et al. [153] compared the effect of the LNG-IUS and a Cu-IUD on menstruation and dysmenorrhea in women with and without adenomyosis and found that the LNG-IUS significantly improved SDys, as well as the characteristics of menstrual bleeding and Hb levels in subjects with adenomyosis. They also observed that acne was significantly increased in LNG-IUS bearers. Over a period of 3 years, Sheng et al. [154] followed 94 women with adenomyosis and moderate or severe dysmenorrhea; they observed that the dysmenorrhea VAS score dropped continuously and significantly from a score of 77.9 ± 14.7 to 11.8 ± 17.9 at 36 months ($p < 0.001$). This drop was accompanied by a significant decrease in the uterine volume, and the overall satisfaction rate for the treatment was 72.5%.

Information is also available on the "frameless" LNG-IUS (FibroPlant) developed by a Belgian Group. In a preliminary trial, Wildemeersch et al. [155] tested the new device in 22 subjects, of whom 8 had primary dysmenorrhea and 10 had secondary dysmenorrhea. All women reported substantially reduced pain, or no pain at all. The overall performance of this system was summarized in 2017, and in subjects with dysmenorrhea, the device was found to be as effective as the classic one [65].

In conclusion, LNG-IUS and frameless devices have been linked to an improvement in dysmenorrhea.

10. Specific Issues

For decades, it has been maintained that intrauterine contraception is contraindicated in adolescents and young and nulliparous women, in spite of evidence to the contrary [156,157].

10.1. Barriers to Use

Buhling et al. [158], in eight European countries plus Canada, evaluated knowledge, attitudes, and beliefs in over 1000 healthcare providers vis-à-vis intrauterine contraception (IUC), concluding that the predominant concerns were nulliparity and pelvic inflammatory disease (PID) for women in general and insertion difficulty and pain, PID, and infertility for nulliparous women; this in spite of the fact that the World Health Organization Medical Eligibility Criteria for IUC lists "nulliparity" under category 2 (benefits outweigh risks) [159]. Focusing on Canada, Hauck and Costescu [160] concluded that to overcome misperceptions about the use of IUC, it is necessary to educate care providers, women, and policy makers.

10.2. Use in Young Women

Back in 2010, a short-term comparative trial [161] showed that at 6 months in adolescent girls (14–18 years old), continuation rates tended to be greater with the LNG-IUS than with the Cu-IUD. In the same year, another investigation [162] reported on 48 adolescents (mean age 15.3 years) bearing the LNG-IUS for over 8 years, mostly because of menorrhagia and dysmenorrhea resistant to oral treatment. In the vast majority (93.4%), there was a significant improvement in their menstrual symptoms.

Clear advantages exist in treatment with the LNG-IUS in adolescents with HMB, dysmenorrhea, and pelvic pain/endometriosis, and, indeed, good results have been reported in young women with AUB, dysmenorrhea, and pelvic pain related to endometriosis [163].

10.3. Safety, Side Effects, and Reasons for Failure

A description of the adverse effects of the LNG-IUS is beyond the scope of this review; the reader may refer to review articles on the subject (e.g., [110,164–166]).

On the other hand, it is perfectly relevant to briefly summarize existing views on the pathophysiological mechanism through which side effects manifest themselves.

Jimenez et al. [167] tried to quantify subendometrial microvascularization and uterine artery blood flow in subjects bearing either the LNG-IUS or the T-Cu 380A. They observed increased subendometrial blood flow in subjects with severe dysmenorrhea and/or AUB after controlling for the device type, age, and parity. However, the pulsatility and resistance indices were not different in these women, leading to the conclusion that measuring these parameters could become a prognostic factor to better evaluate the risk of developing dysmenorrhea and/or bleeding after device insertion.

An attempt to identify factors associated with the failure of the LNG-IUS in controlling HMB was made by Beelen et al. [128], who used data from a cohort of women aged 34 years and older, without intracavitary pathology and without plans for future children, treated with the device and suffering from AUB. A multivariable analysis showed younger age

(age below 45) (adjusted RR = 1.51; 95% CI = 1.10–2.09; p = 0.012) and severe dysmenorrhea (adjusted RR = 1.36; 95% CI = 1.01–1.82; p = 0.041) to be associated with a higher risk of discontinuation.

11. Conclusions

Over the last quarter of a century, evidence has been accumulating showing that the LNG-IUS, in all of its variants, represents a useful tool to combat both AUB and dysmenorrhea in women of all ages. Almost all published trials have reported improvements for both conditions. Perhaps the most important mechanism of action of the LNG-IUS is attributable to its ability to induce amenorrhea, which effectively eliminates HMB and dysmenorrhea. While new generations of therapeutics are now becoming available, the low cost and ease of use make the LNG-IUS very attractive, especially when contraception is also desired. Still, for large uteri, the LNG-IUS may be less effective, and there has been limited level I data on its efficacy in treating endometrial-polyp-induced HMB. Regardless, the LNG-IUS is and is expected to remain, in the foreseeable future, a viable option for treating AUB and dysmenorrhea.

Author Contributions: P.B. prepared the first draft, selected the figures and oversaw the revisions; S.-W.G. and M.H. added to the first draft, completing a number of sections. G.B. conceived the idea, prepared the TOC and reviewed the final text. All authors have read and agreed to the published version of the manuscript.

Funding: This research received no external funding.

Institutional Review Board Statement: Not applicable.

Informed Consent Statement: Not applicable.

Data Availability Statement: No unpublished data from the Authors were reported.

Conflicts of Interest: The authors declare no conflict of interest.

References

1. Critchley, H.O.D.; Maybin, J.A.; Armstrong, G.M.; Williams, A.R.W. Physiology of the Endometrium and Regulation of Menstruation. *Physiol. Rev.* **2020**, *100*, 1149–1179. [CrossRef] [PubMed]
2. Davis, E.; Sparzak, P.B. *Abnormal Uterine Bleeding*; StatPearls: Treasure Island, FL, USA, 2022.
3. Ju, H.; Jones, M.; Mishra, G. The Prevalence and Risk Factors of Dysmenorrhea. *Epidemiol. Rev.* **2014**, *36*, 104–113. [CrossRef] [PubMed]
4. Tadese, M.; Kassa, A.; Muluneh, A.A.; Altaye, G. Prevalence of dysmenorrhoea, associated risk factors and its relationship with academic performance among graduating female university students in Ethiopia: A cross-sectional study. *BMJ Open* **2021**, *11*, e043814. [CrossRef] [PubMed]
5. Munro, M.G.; Critchley, H.O.; Fraser, I.S.; The FIGO Menstrual Disorders Committee. The two FIGO systems for normal and abnormal uterine bleeding symptoms and classification of causes of abnormal uterine bleeding in the reproductive years: 2018 revisions. *Int. J. Gynecol. Obstet.* **2018**, *143*, 393–408, Erratum in *Int. J. Gynecol. Obstet.* **2019**, *144*, 237. [CrossRef] [PubMed]
6. Munro, M.G.; Balen, A.H.; Cho, S.; Critchley, H.; Díaz, I.; Ferriani, R.; Henry, L.; Mocanu, E.; van der Spuy, Z.M. FIGO Committee on Menstrual Disorders and Related Health Impacts; FIGO Committee on Reproductive Medicine, Endocrinology, and Infertility. The FIGO Ovulatory Disorders Classification System. *Hum. Reprod.* **2022**, deac180, *Advance online publication*. [CrossRef]
7. Bradley, L.D.; Gueye, N.-A. The medical management of abnormal uterine bleeding in reproductive-aged women. *Am. J. Obstet. Gynecol.* **2016**, *214*, 31–44. [CrossRef] [PubMed]
8. McKenna, K.A.; Fogleman, C.D. Dysmenorrhea. *Am. Fam. Physician* **2021**, *104*, 164–170.
9. Smith, R.P. *Dysmenorrhea and Menorrhagia: A Clinician's Guide*; Springer Nature: London, UK; Berlin/Heidelberg, Germany, 2018.
10. ACOG Practice Bulletin No. 110: Noncontraceptive Uses of Hormonal Contraceptives. *Obstet. Gynecol.* **2010**, *115*, 206–218. [CrossRef]
11. Armstrong, C. ACOG Recommendations on Emergency Contraception. *Am. Fam. Physician* **2010**, *82*, 1278.
12. Warner, P.E.; Critchley, H.O.; Lumsden, M.A.; Campbell-Brown, M.; Douglas, A.; Murray, G. Menorrhagia II: Is the 80-mL blood loss criterion useful in management of complaint of menorrhagia? *Am. J. Obstet. Gynecol.* **2004**, *190*, 1224–1229. [CrossRef]
13. Warner, P.E.; Critchley, H.O.; Lumsden, M.A.; Campbell-Brown, M.; Douglas, A.; Murray, G.D. Menorrhagia I: Measured blood loss, clinical features, and outcome in women with heavy periods: A survey with follow-up data. *Am. J. Obstet. Gynecol.* **2004**, *190*, 1216–1223. [CrossRef]

14. Hallberg, L.; Högdahl, A.-M.; Nilsson, L.; Rybo, G. Menstrual Blood Loss–A Population Study: Variation at different ages and attempts to define normality. *Acta Obstet. Gynecol. Scand.* **1966**, *45*, 320–351. [CrossRef] [PubMed]
15. NICE. *NICE Guideline [NG88]: Heavy Menstrual Bleeding: Assessment and Management*; National Institute for Health and Care Excellence: London, UK, 2018.
16. American College of Obstetricians and Gynecologists. Management of abnormal uterine bleeding associated with ovulatory dysfunction. *Obstet. Gynecol.* **2013**, *122*, 176–185. [CrossRef]
17. Matteson, K.A.; Rahn, D.D.; Wheeler, T.L., 2nd; Casiano, E.A.; Siddiqui, N.Y.; Harvie, H.S.; Mamik, M.M.; Balk, E.M.; Sung, V.W.; Society of Gynecologic Surgeons Systematic Review Group. Nonsurgical Management of Heavy Menstrual Bleeding: A Systematic Review. *Obstet. Gynecol.* **2013**, *121*, 632–643. [CrossRef] [PubMed]
18. Munro, M.; Critchley, H.; Fraser, I. Research and clinical management for women with abnormal uterine bleeding in the reproductive years: More than PALM-COEIN. *BJOG Int. J. Obstet. Gynaecol.* **2017**, *124*, 185–189. [CrossRef] [PubMed]
19. Heikinheimo, O.; Fraser, I. The current status of hormonal therapies for heavy menstrual bleeding. *Best Pract. Res. Clin. Obstet. Gynaecol.* **2017**, *40*, 111–120. [CrossRef]
20. Davies, J.; Kadir, R.A. Heavy menstrual bleeding: An update on management. *Thromb. Res.* **2017**, *151* (Suppl. 1), S70–S77. [CrossRef]
21. Rodriguez, M.B.; Lethaby, A.; Farquhar, C. Non-steroidal anti-inflammatory drugs for heavy menstrual bleeding. *Cochrane Database Syst. Rev.* **2019**, *9*, CD000400. [CrossRef]
22. Lethaby, A.; Augood, C.; Duckitt, K.; Farquhar, C. Nonsteroidal anti-inflammatory drugs for heavy menstrual bleeding. *Cochrane Database Syst. Rev.* **2007**, CD000400. [CrossRef]
23. Rodriguez, M.B.; Lethaby, A.; Jordan, V. Progestogen-releasing intrauterine systems for heavy menstrual bleeding. *Cochrane Database Syst. Rev.* **2020**, *6*, CD002126. [CrossRef]
24. Iacovides, S.; Avidon, I.; Baker, F.C. What we know about primary dysmenorrhea today: A critical review. *Hum. Reprod. Update* **2015**, *21*, 762–778. [CrossRef]
25. NICE, National Institute for Health Care Excellence. *Dysmenorrhoea*; NICE: London, UK, 2020.
26. ACOG Committee Opinion No. 760: Dysmenorrhea and Endometriosis in the Adolescent. *Obstet. Gynecol.* **2018**, *132*, e249–e258. [CrossRef]
27. Margatho, D.; Carvalho, N.M.; Eloy, L.; Bahamondes, L. Assessment of biomarkers in women with endometriosis-associated pain using the ENG contraceptive implant or the 52 mg LNG-IUS: A non-inferiority randomised clinical trial. *Eur. J. Contracept. Reprod. Health Care* **2018**, *23*, 344–350. [CrossRef] [PubMed]
28. Carvalho, N.; Margatho, D.; Cursino, K.; Benetti-Pinto, C.L.; Bahamondes, L. Control of endometriosis-associated pain with etonogestrel-releasing contraceptive implant and 52-mg levonorgestrel-releasing intrauterine system: Randomized clinical trial. *Fertil. Steril.* **2018**, *110*, 1129–1136. [CrossRef] [PubMed]
29. Margatho, D.; Carvalho, N.M.; Bahamondes, L. Endometriosis-associated pain scores and biomarkers in users of the etonogestrel-releasing subdermal implant or the 52-mg levonorgestrel-releasing intrauterine system for up to 24 months. *Eur. J. Contracept. Reprod. Health Care* **2020**, *25*, 133–140. [CrossRef] [PubMed]
30. Doyle, L.L.; Clewe, T.H. Preliminary studies on the effect of hormone-releasing intrauterine devices. *Am. J. Obstet. Gynecol.* **1968**, *101*, 564–568. [CrossRef]
31. Strycker, J.C.; Doyle, L.L.; Clewe, T.H.; Lippes, J. Silastic Lippes loop with crystalline Provera. *Excerpta Med. Int. Congr. Ser.* **1971**, *246*, 100.
32. Scommegna, A.; Pandya, G.N.; Christ, M.; Lee, A.W.; Cohen, M.R. Intrauterine Administration of Progesterone by a Slow Releasing Device. *Fertil. Steril.* **1970**, *21*, 201–210. [CrossRef]
33. Pandya, G.N.; Scommegna, A. Intrauterine progesterone releasing device—A clinical trial. *Excerpta Med. Int. Congr. Ser.* **1972**.
34. Pharriss, B.B.; Erickson, R.; Bashaw, J.; Hoff, S.; Place, V.A.; Zaffaroni, A. Progestasert: A Uterine Therapeutic System for Long-term Contraception: I. Philosophy and Clinical Efficacy. *Fertil. Steril.* **1974**, *25*, 915–921. [CrossRef]
35. Burnhill, M.S. The rise and fall and rise of the IUD. *Am. J. Gynecol. Health* **1989**, *3*, 6–10.
36. Snowden, R. The Progestasert and ectopic pregnancy. *BMJ* **1977**, *2*, 1600–1601. [CrossRef]
37. Hagenfeldt, K.; Landgren, B.-M. Contraception by intrauterine release of progesterone—Effects on endometrial trace elements, enzymes and steroids. *J. Steroid Biochem.* **1975**, *6*, 895–898. [CrossRef]
38. Hagenfeldt, K.; Landgren, B.-M.; Edström, K.; Johannisson, E. Biochemical and morphological changes in the human endometrium induced by the progestasert device. *Contraception* **1977**, *16*, 183–197. [CrossRef]
39. Shaw, S., Jr.; Macaulay, L.; Aznar, R.; Gonzalez-Angulo, A.; Roy, S. Effects of a progesterone-releasing intrauterine contraceptive device on endometrial blood vessels: A morphometric study. *Am. J. Obstet. Gynecol.* **1981**, *141*, 821–827. [CrossRef]
40. Ermin, M.; Carpino, F.; Petrozza, V.; Benagiano, G. Distribution and effect on the endometrium of progesterone released from a progestasert device. *Hum. Reprod.* **1989**, *4*, 221–228. [CrossRef] [PubMed]
41. Nilsson, C.; Johansson, E.D.; Jackanicz, T.M.; Luukkainen, T. Biodegradable polylactate as a steroid-releasing polymer: Intrauterine administration of d-norgestrel. *Am. J. Obstet. Gynecol.* **1975**, *122*, 90–95. [CrossRef]
42. Nilsson, C.G.; Johansson, E.D.B.; Luukkainen, T. A d-norgestrel-releasing IUD. *Contraception* **1976**, *13*, 503–514. [CrossRef]
43. Nilsson, C.G. Comparative quantitation of menstrual blood loss with a d-norgestrel-releasing IUD and a Nova-T-copper device. *Contraception* **1977**, *15*, 379–387. [CrossRef]

44. Nilsson, C.G.; Luukkainen, T.; Arko, H. Endometrial Morphology of Women Using A d-Norgestrel-Releasing Intrauterine Device. *Fertil. Steril.* **1978**, *29*, 397–401. [CrossRef]
45. Luukkainen, T.; Allonen, H.; Haukkamaa, M.; Lähteenmäki, P.; Nilsson, C.G.; Toivonen, J. Five years' experience with levonorgestrel-releasing IUDs. *Contraception* **1986**, *33*, 139–148. [CrossRef]
46. FDA. Mirena (Levonorgestrel-Releasing Intrauterine System). Available online: https://www.accessdata.fda.gov/drugsatfda_docs/label/2008/021225s019lbl.pdf (accessed on 9 August 2022).
47. Mirena. Package Insert. Bayer. 2022. Available online: https://www.accessdata.fda.gov/drugsatfda_docs/label/2022/021225s043lbl.pdf (accessed on 9 August 2022).
48. Jensen, J.T.; Reinecke, I.; Lukkari-Lax, E.; Hofmann, B.M. Estimating In Vivo Levonorgestrel Release Rate and Exposure Over Eight Years with Levonorgestrel Releasing Intrauterine System 52 mg Use With Population Pharmacokinetic Approach [A03]. *Obstet. Gynecol. (Ann Clin Scient Meeting Abst Suppl.)* **2022**, *139*, 1S. [CrossRef]
49. Faundes, A.; Alvarez, F.; Brache, V.; Tejada, A. The role of the levonorgestrel intrauterine device in the prevention and treatment of iron deficiency anemia during fertility regulation. *Int. J. Gynecol. Obstet.* **1988**, *26*, 429–433. [CrossRef]
50. Andersson, J.K.; Rybo, G. Levonorgestrel-releasing intrauterine device in the treatment of menorrhagia. *BJOG Int. J. Obstet. Gynaecol.* **1990**, *97*, 690–694. [CrossRef] [PubMed]
51. Milsom, I.; Andersson, K.; Andersch, B.; Rybo, G. A comparison of flurbiprofen, tranexamic acid, and a levonorgestrel-releasing intrauterine contraceptive device in the treatment of idiopathic menorrhagia. *Am. J. Obstet. Gynecol.* **1991**, *164*, 879–883. [CrossRef]
52. Luukkainen, T. The levonorgestrel intrauterine system: Therapeutic aspects. *Steroids* **2000**, *65*, 699–702. [CrossRef]
53. Pakarinen, P.; Toivonen, J.; Luukkainen, T. Therapeutic Use of the LNG IUS, and Counseling. *Semin. Reprod. Med.* **2001**, *19*, 365–372. [CrossRef]
54. Varma, R.; Sinha, D.; Gupta, J.K. Non-contraceptive uses of levonorgestrel-releasing hormone system (LNG-IUS)—A systematic enquiry and overview. *Eur. J. Obstet. Gynecol. Reprod. Biol.* **2006**, *125*, 9–28. [CrossRef]
55. Bednarek, P.H.; Jensen, J. Safety, efficacy and patient acceptability of the contraceptive and non-contraceptive uses of the LNG-IUS. *Int. J. Women's Health* **2009**, *1*, 45–58. [CrossRef]
56. Rose, S.; Chaudhari, A.; Peterson, C.M. Mirena (Levonorgestrel intrauterine system): A successful novel drug delivery option in contraception. *Adv. Drug Deliv. Rev.* **2009**, *61*, 808–812. [CrossRef]
57. Fraser, I.S. Non-contraceptive health benefits of intrauterine hormonal systems. *Contraception* **2010**, *82*, 396–403. [CrossRef]
58. Heikinheimo, O.; Gemzell-Danielsson, K. Emerging indications for the levonorgestrel-releasing intrauterine system (LNG-IUS). *Acta Obstet. Gynecol. Scand.* **2012**, *91*, 3–9. [CrossRef]
59. Sabbioni, L.; Petraglia, F.; Luisi, S. Non-contraceptive benefits of intrauterine levonorgestrel administration: Why not? *Gynecol. Endocrinol.* **2017**, *33*, 822–829. [CrossRef]
60. Cristobal, I.; Lete, L.I.; de la Viuda, E.; Perulero, N.; Arbat, A.; Canals, I. One year quality of life measured with SEC-QoL in levonorgestrel 52 mg IUS users. *Contraception* **2016**, *93*, 367–371. [CrossRef]
61. Gemzell-Danielsson, K.; Apter, D.; Dermout, S.; Faustmann, T.; Rosen, K.; Schmelter, T.; Merz, M.; Nelson, A. Evaluation of a new, low-dose levonorgestrel intrauterine contraceptive system over 5 years of use. *Eur. J. Obstet. Gynecol. Reprod. Biol.* **2017**, *210*, 22–28. [CrossRef] [PubMed]
62. Nelson, A.L. Levonorgestrel-Releasing Intrauterine System (LNG-IUS 12) for Prevention of Pregnancy for Up to Five Years. *Expert Rev. Clin. Pharmacol.* **2017**, *10*, 833–842. [CrossRef] [PubMed]
63. Gemzell-Danielsson, K.; Buhling, K.J.; Dermout, S.M.; Lukkari-Lax, E.; Montegriffo, E.; Apter, D. A Phase III, single-arm study of LNG-IUS 8, a low-dose levonorgestrel intrauterine contraceptive system (total content 13.5 mg) in postmenarcheal adolescents. *Contraception* **2016**, *93*, 507–512. [CrossRef]
64. Wildemeersch, D.; Jandi, S.; Pett, A.; Nolte, K.; Hasskamp, T.; Vrijens, M. Use of frameless intrauterine devices and systems in young nulliparous and adolescent women: Results of a multicenter study. *Int. J. Women's Health* **2014**, *6*, 727–734. [CrossRef]
65. Yang, H.; Wang, S.; Fu, X.; Lan, R.; Gong, H. Effect of modified levonorgestrel-releasing intrauterine system in human adenomyosis with heavy menstrual bleeding. *J. Obstet. Gynaecol. Res.* **2022**, *48*, 161–168. [CrossRef] [PubMed]
66. Wildemeersch, D.; Andrade, A.; Goldstuck, N.D.; Hasskamp, T.; Jackers, G. Intrauterine levonorgestrel delivery with frameless fibrous delivery system: Review of clinical experience. *Int. J. Women's Health* **2017**, *9*, 49–58. [CrossRef] [PubMed]
67. Ilyin, A.B.; Khasanov, A.A.; Suturina, L.V.; Borisova, N.I.; Reshetov, Z.S.; Foidart, J.-M.; Déri, J.A.; Tóth, V. Comparison of two levonorgestrel-releasing intrauterine systems for the treatment of heavy menstrual bleeding: A randomised, controlled, phase 3 trial. *Eur. J. Contracept. Reprod. Health Care* **2021**, *26*, 491–498. [CrossRef]
68. WHO. Available online: https://www.who.int/publications/i/item/9789240021730 (accessed on 9 August 2022).
69. Creinin, M.; Kohn, J.E.; Tang, J.H.; Serna, T.B.; Society of Family Planning Clinical Affairs Committee. Society of Family Planning Committee statement on IUD nomenclature. *Contraception* **2022**, *106*, 1–2. [CrossRef] [PubMed]
70. Munro, M.G.; Critchley, H.O.; Broder, M.S.; Fraser, I.S.; FIGO Working Group on Menstrual Disorders. FIGO classification system (PALM-COEIN) for causes of abnormal uterine bleeding in nongravid women of reproductive age. *Int. J. Gynecol. Obstet.* **2011**, *113*, 3–13. [CrossRef] [PubMed]
71. Critchley, H.O.D.; Jones, R.L.; Lea, R.G.; Drudy, T.A.; Kelly, R.W.; Williams, A.R.W.; Baird, D.T. Role of Inflammatory Mediators in Human Endometrium during Progesterone Withdrawal and Early Pregnancy. *J. Clin. Endocrinol. Metab.* **1999**, *84*, 240–248. [CrossRef] [PubMed]

72. Sugino, N.; Karube-Harada, A.; Taketani, T.; Sakata, A.; Nakamura, Y. Withdrawal of Ovarian Steroids Stimulates Prostaglandin F2α Production Through Nuclear Factor-κB Activation via Oxygen Radicals in Human Endometrial Stromal Cells: Potential Relevance to Menstruation. *J. Reprod. Dev.* **2004**, *50*, 215–225. [CrossRef] [PubMed]
73. Critchley, H.O.D.; Osei, J.; Henderson, T.A.; Boswell, L.; Sales, K.; Jabbour, H.N.; Hirani, N. Hypoxia-Inducible Factor-1α Expression in Human Endometrium and Its Regulation by Prostaglandin E-Series Prostanoid Receptor 2 (EP2). *Endocrinology* **2006**, *147*, 744–753. [CrossRef]
74. Maybin, J.A.; Hirani, N.; Jabbour, H.N.; Critchley, H.O. Novel Roles for Hypoxia and Prostaglandin E2 in the Regulation of IL-8 During Endometrial Repair. *Am. J. Pathol.* **2011**, *178*, 1245–1256. [CrossRef]
75. Maybin, J.A.; Murray, A.A.; Saunders, P.T.K.; Hirani, N.; Carmeliet, P.; Critchley, H.O.D. Hypoxia and hypoxia inducible factor-1α are required for normal endometrial repair during menstruation. *Nat. Commun.* **2018**, *9*, 295. [CrossRef]
76. Munro, M.G. Classification of menstrual bleeding disorders. *Rev. Endocr. Metab. Disord.* **2012**, *13*, 225–234. [CrossRef]
77. Huang, Q.; Liu, X.; Critchley, H.; Fu, Z.; Guo, S. How does the extent of fibrosis in adenomyosis lesions contribute to heavy menstrual bleeding? *Reprod. Med. Biol.* **2022**, *21*, e12442. [CrossRef]
78. Huang, X.; Yang, N.; Fiore, V.F.; Barker, T.H.; Sun, Y.; Morris, S.W.; Ding, Q.; Thannickal, V.J.; Zhou, Y. Matrix Stiffness–Induced Myofibroblast Differentiation Is Mediated by Intrinsic Mechanotransduction. *Am. J. Respir. Cell Mol. Biol.* **2012**, *47*, 340–348. [CrossRef]
79. Marinković, A.; Mih, J.D.; Park, J.-A.; Liu, F.; Tschumperlin, D.J. Improved throughput traction microscopy reveals pivotal role for matrix stiffness in fibroblast contractility and TGF-β responsiveness. *Am. J. Physiol.-Lung Cell. Mol. Physiol.* **2012**, *303*, L169–L180. [CrossRef] [PubMed]
80. Giménez, A.; Duch, P.; Puig, M.; Gabasa, M.; Xaubet, A.; Alcaraz, J. Dysregulated Collagen Homeostasis by Matrix Stiffening and TGF-β1 in Fibroblasts from Idiopathic Pulmonary Fibrosis Patients: Role of FAK/Akt. *Int. J. Mol. Sci.* **2017**, *18*, 2431. [CrossRef] [PubMed]
81. Berhan, A.; Harris, T.; Jaffar, J.; Jativa, F.; Langenbach, S.; Lönnstedt, I.; Alhamdoosh, M.; Ng, M.; Lee, P.; Westall, G.; et al. Cellular Microenvironment Stiffness Regulates Eicosanoid Production and Signaling Pathways. *Am. J. Respir. Cell Mol. Biol.* **2020**, *63*, 819–830. [CrossRef] [PubMed]
82. Liu, F.; Mih, J.D.; Shea, B.S.; Kho, A.T.; Sharif, A.S.; Tager, A.M.; Tschumperlin, D.J. Feedback amplification of fibrosis through matrix stiffening and COX-2 suppression. *J. Cell Biol.* **2010**, *190*, 693–706. [CrossRef] [PubMed]
83. Marinković, A.; Liu, F.; Tschumperlin, D.J. Matrices of Physiologic Stiffness Potently Inactivate Idiopathic Pulmonary Fibrosis Fibroblasts. *Am. J. Respir. Cell Mol. Biol.* **2013**, *48*, 422–430. [CrossRef]
84. Bärnthaler, T.; Theiler, A.; Zabini, D.; Trautmann, S.; Stacher-Priehse, E.; Lanz, I.; Klepetko, W.; Sinn, K.; Flick, H.; Scheidl, S.; et al. Inhibiting eicosanoid degradation exerts antifibrotic effects in a pulmonary fibrosis mouse model and human tissue. *J. Allergy Clin. Immunol.* **2020**, *145*, 818–833.e11. [CrossRef]
85. Huang, Q.; Liu, X.; Guo, S. Higher fibrotic content of endometriotic lesions is associated with diminished prostaglandin E2 signaling. *Reprod. Med. Biol.* **2022**, *21*, e12423. [CrossRef]
86. Ishiwata, I.; Ishiwata, C.; Ishikawa, H. Effects of Estradiol-17β and Progesterone on Cell Proliferation and Differentiation of the Human Endometrial Carcinoma Cell Line (HHUA) in Vitro. *Asia-Oceania J. Obstet. Gynaecol.* **1984**, *10*, 531–538. [CrossRef]
87. White, J.; Sullivan, M.; Patel, L.; Croxtall, J.; D'Arcangues, C.; Belsey, E.; Elder, M. Prostaglandin production in human endometrium following continuous exposure to low-dose levonorgestrel released from a vaginal ring. *Contraception* **1991**, *43*, 401–412. [CrossRef]
88. Mueller, A.; Siemer, J.; Schreiner, S.; Koesztner, H.; Hoffmann, I.; Binder, H.; Beckmann, M.; Dittrich, R. Role of estrogen and progesterone in the regulation of uterine peristalsis: Results from perfused non-pregnant swine uteri. *Hum. Reprod.* **2006**, *21*, 1863–1868. [CrossRef]
89. Chen, C.-C.; Montalbano, A.P.; Hussain, I.; Lee, W.-R.; Mendelson, C.R. The transcriptional repressor GATAD2B mediates progesterone receptor suppression of myometrial contractile gene expression. *J. Biol. Chem.* **2017**, *292*, 12560–12575. [CrossRef] [PubMed]
90. Peavey, M.C.; Wu, S.-P.; Li, R.; Liu, J.; Emery, O.M.; Wang, T.; Zhou, L.; Wetendorf, M.; Yallampalli, C.; Gibbons, W.E.; et al. Progesterone receptor isoform B regulates the *Oxtr-Plcl2-Trpc3* pathway to suppress uterine contractility. *Proc. Natl. Acad. Sci. USA* **2021**, *118*, e2011643118. [CrossRef] [PubMed]
91. Hardy, D.B.; Janowski, B.A.; Corey, D.R.; Mendelson, C. Progesterone Receptor Plays a Major Antiinflammatory Role in Human Myometrial Cells by Antagonism of Nuclear Factor-κB Activation of Cyclooxygenase 2 Expression. *Mol. Endocrinol.* **2006**, *20*, 2724–2733. [CrossRef] [PubMed]
92. Elovitz, M.A.; Ascher-Landsberg, J.; Saunders, T.; Phillippe, M. The mechanisms underlying the stimulatory effects of thrombin on myometrial smooth muscle. *Am. J. Obstet. Gynecol.* **2000**, *183*, 674–681. [CrossRef]
93. Elovitz, M.; Saunders, T.; Ascher-Landsberg, J.; Phillippe, M. Effects of thrombin on myometrial contractions in vitro and in vivo. *Am. J. Obstet. Gynecol.* **2000**, *183*, 799–804. [CrossRef]
94. Nie, J.; Lu, Y.; Liu, X.; Guo, S.-W. Immunoreactivity of progesterone receptor isoform B, nuclear factor κB, and IκBα in adenomyosis. *Fertil. Steril.* **2009**, *92*, 886–889. [CrossRef]
95. Attia, G.R.; Zeitoun, K.; Edwards, D.; Johns, A.; Carr, B.R.; Bulun, S.E. Progesterone Receptor Isoform A But Not B Is Expressed in Endometriosis1. *J. Clin. Endocrinol. Metab.* **2000**, *85*, 2897–2902. [CrossRef]

96. Montgomery, B.E.; Daum, G.S.; Dunton, C.J. Endometrial Hyperplasia: A Review. *Obstet. Gynecol. Surv.* **2004**, *59*, 368–378. [CrossRef]
97. Kim, J.; Chapman-Davis, E. Role of Progesterone in Endometrial Cancer. *Semin. Reprod. Med.* **2010**, *28*, 81–90. [CrossRef]
98. Mittal, K.; Schwartz, L.; Goswami, S.; Demopoulos, R. Estrogen and Progesterone Receptor Expression in Endometrial Polyps. *Int. J. Gynecol. Pathol.* **1996**, *15*, 345–348. [CrossRef]
99. Feng, M.; Zhang, T.; Ma, H. Progesterone ameliorates the endometrial polyp by modulating the signaling pathway of Wnt and β-catenin via regulating the expression of H19 and miR-152. *J. Cell. Biochem.* **2019**, *120*, 10164–10174. [CrossRef] [PubMed]
100. Wu, Y.; Strawn, E.; Basir, Z.; Halverson, G.; Guo, S.-W. Promoter Hypermethylation of Progesterone Receptor Isoform B (PR-B) in Endometriosis. *Epigenetics* **2006**, *1*, 106–111. [CrossRef] [PubMed]
101. Nie, J.; Liu, X.; Guo, S.-W. Promoter Hypermethylation of Progesterone Receptor Isoform B (PR-B) in Adenomyosis and Its Rectification by a Histone Deacetylase Inhibitor and a Demethylation Agent. *Reprod. Sci.* **2010**, *17*, 995–1005. [CrossRef] [PubMed]
102. Inoue, S.; Hirota, Y.; Ueno, T.; Fukui, Y.; Yoshida, E.; Hayashi, T.; Kojima, S.; Takeyama, R.; Hashimoto, T.; Kiyono, T.; et al. Uterine adenomyosis is an oligoclonal disorder associated with KRAS mutations. *Nat. Commun.* **2019**, *10*, 5785. [CrossRef] [PubMed]
103. Ishikawa, H.; Ishi, K.; Serna, V.A.; Kakazu, R.; Bulun, S.E.; Kurita, T. Progesterone Is Essential for Maintenance and Growth of Uterine Leiomyoma. *Endocrinology* **2010**, *151*, 2433–2442. [CrossRef] [PubMed]
104. Kim, J.J.; Sefton, E.C. The role of progesterone signaling in the pathogenesis of uterine leiomyoma. *Mol. Cell. Endocrinol.* **2012**, *358*, 223–231. [CrossRef] [PubMed]
105. Islam, S.; Ciavattini, A.; Petraglia, F.; Castellucci, M.; Ciarmela, P. Extracellular matrix in uterine leiomyoma pathogenesis: A potential target for future therapeutics. *Hum. Reprod. Updat.* **2018**, *24*, 59–85. [CrossRef] [PubMed]
106. Venkatachalam, S.; Bagratee, J.; Moodley, J. Medical management of uterine fibroids with medroxyprogesterone acetate (Depo Provera): A pilot study. *J. Obstet. Gynaecol.* **2004**, *24*, 798–800. [CrossRef]
107. Johnson, N.; Fletcher, H.; Reid, M. Depo medroxyprogesterone acetate (DMPA) therapy for uterine myomata prior to surgery. *Int. J. Gynecol. Obstet.* **2004**, *85*, 174–176. [CrossRef]
108. Harmon, Q.; Baird, D. Use of depot medroxyprogesterone acetate and prevalent leiomyoma in young African American women. *Hum. Reprod.* **2015**, *30*, 1499–1504. [CrossRef]
109. Benagiano, G.; Morini, A.; Aleandri, V.; Piccinno, F.; Primiero, F.M.; Abbondante, G.; Elkind-Hirsch, K. Sequential Gn-RH superagonist and medroxyprogesterone acetate treatment of uterine leiomyomata. *Int. J. Gynecol. Obstet.* **1990**, *33*, 333–343. [CrossRef]
110. Palomba, S.; Sena, T.; Morelli, M.; Noia, R.; Zullo, F.; Mastrantonio, P. Effect of different doses of progestin on uterine leiomyomas in postmenopausal women. *Eur. J. Obstet. Gynecol. Reprod. Biol.* **2002**, *102*, 199–201. [CrossRef]
111. Carr, B.R.; Marshburn, P.B.; Weatherall, P.T.; Bradshaw, K.D.; Breslau, N.A.; Byrd, W.; Roark, M.; Steinkampf, M.P. An evaluation of the effect of gonadotropin-releasing hormone analogs and medroxyprogesterone acetate on uterine leiomyomata volume by magnetic resonance imaging: A prospective, randomized, double blind, placebo-controlled, crossover trial. *J. Clin. Endocrinol. Metab.* **1993**, *76*, 1217–1223. [CrossRef] [PubMed]
112. Friedman, A.J.; Daly, M.; Juneau-Norcross, M.; Rein, M.S.; Fine, C.; Gleason, R.; LeBoff, M. A prospective, randomized trial of gonadotropin-releasing hormone agonist plus estrogen-progestin or progestin "add-back" regimens for women with leiomyomata uteri. *J. Clin. Endocrinol. Metab.* **1993**, *76*, 1439–1445. [CrossRef]
113. Teal, S.B.; Turok, D.; Chen, B.A.; Kimble, T.; Olariu, A.I.; Creinin, M.D. Five-Year Contraceptive Efficacy and Safety of a Levonorgestrel 52-mg Intrauterine System. *Obstet. Gynecol.* **2019**, *133*, 63–70. [CrossRef]
114. Magalhaes, J.; Ferreira-Filho, E.S.; Soares-Junior, J.M.; Baracat, E.C. Uterine volume, menstrual patterns, and contraceptive outcomes in users of the levonorgestrel-releasing intrauterine system: A cohort study with a five-year follow-up. *Eur. J. Obstet. Gynecol. Reprod. Biol.* **2022**, *276*, 56–62. [CrossRef]
115. Brosens, I.A. Endometriosis—A disease because it is characterized by bleeding. *Am. J. Obstet. Gynecol.* **1997**, *176*, 263–267. [CrossRef]
116. Fedele, L.; Bianchi, S.; Raffaelli, R.; Portuese, A.; Dorta, M. Treatment of adenomyosis-associated menorrhagia with a levonorgestrel-releasing intrauterine device. *Fertil. Steril.* **1997**, *68*, 426–429. [CrossRef]
117. Barrington, J.W.; Bowen-Simpkins, P. The levonorgestrel intrauterine system in the management of menorrhagia. *BJOG Int. J. Obstet. Gynaecol.* **1997**, *104*, 614–616. [CrossRef]
118. Peng, F.-S.; Wu, M.-Y.; Yang, J.-H.; Chen, S.-U.; Ho, H.-N.; Yang, Y.-S. Insertion of the Mirena Intrauterine System for Treatment of Adenomyosis-Associated Menorrhagia: A Novel Method. *Taiwan. J. Obstet. Gynecol.* **2010**, *49*, 160–164. [CrossRef]
119. Uysal, A.; Taner, C.E.; Mun, S.; Uysal, F.; Celimli, F.H. Use of a levonorgestrel-releasing intrauterine device in the treatment of adenomyosis associated heavy menstrual bleeding. *J. Pak. Med. Assoc.* **2013**, *63*, 1349–1352.
120. Grigorieva, V.; Chen-Mok, M.; Tarasova, M.; Mikhailov, A. Use of a levonorgestrel-releasing intrauterine system to treat bleeding related to uterine leiomyomas. *Fertil. Steril.* **2003**, *79*, 1194–1198. [CrossRef]
121. Mercorio, F.; De Simone, R.; Di Spiezio Sardo, A.; Cerrota, G.; Bifulco, G.; Vanacore, F.; Nappi, C. The effect of a levonorgestrel-releasing intrauterine device in the treatment of myoma-related menorrhagia. *Contraception* **2003**, *67*, 277–280. [CrossRef]
122. Magalhães, J.; Aldrighi, J.M.; de Lima, G.R. Uterine volume and menstrual patterns in users of the levonorgestrel-releasing intrauterine system with idiopathic menorrhagia or menorrhagia due to leiomyomas. *Contraception* **2007**, *75*, 193–198. [CrossRef] [PubMed]

123. Naki, M.M.; Tekcan, C.; Ozcan, N.; Cebi, M. Levonorgestrel-releasing intrauterine device insertion ameliorates leiomyoma-dependent menorrhagia among women of reproductive age without a significant regression in the uterine and leiomyoma volumes. *Fertil. Steril.* **2010**, *94*, 371–374. [CrossRef]
124. Socolov, D.; Blidaru, I.; Tamba, B.; Miron, N.; Boiculese, V.L.; Socolov, R. Levonorgestrel releasing-intrauterine system for the treatment of menorrhagia and/or frequent irregular uterine bleeding associated with uterine leiomyoma. *Eur. J. Contracept. Reprod. Health Care* **2011**, *16*, 480–487. [CrossRef]
125. Senol, T.; Kahramanoglu, I.; Dogan, Y.; Baktiroglu, M.; Karateke, A.; Suer, N. Levonorgestrel-releasing intrauterine device use as an alternative to surgical therapy for uterine leiomyoma. *Clin. Exp. Obstet. Gynecol.* **2015**, *42*, 224–227. [CrossRef]
126. Kaunitz, A.M.; Bissonnette, F.; Monteiro, I.; Lukkari-Lax, E.; Muysers, C.; Jensen, J. Levonorgestrel-Releasing Intrauterine System or Medroxyprogesterone for Heavy Menstrual Bleeding: A Randomized Controlled Trial. *Obstet. Gynecol.* **2010**, *116*, 625–632. [CrossRef] [PubMed]
127. Wildemeersch, D.; Schacht, E. Treatment of menorrhagia with a novel 'frameless' intrauterine levonorgestrel-releasing drug delivery system: A pilot study. *Eur. J. Contracept. Reprod. Health Care* **2001**, *6*, 93–101. [CrossRef] [PubMed]
128. Kaislasuo, J.; Heikinheimo, O.; Lähteenmäki, P.; Suhonen, S. Menstrual characteristics and ultrasonographic uterine cavity measurements predict bleeding and pain in nulligravid women using intrauterine contraception. *Hum. Reprod.* **2015**, *30*, 1580–1588. [CrossRef] [PubMed]
129. Beelen, P.; Brink, M.J.V.D.; Herman, M.C.; Geomini, P.M.; Duijnhoven, R.G.; Bongers, M.Y. Predictive factors for failure of the levonorgestrel releasing intrauterine system in women with heavy menstrual bleeding. *BMC Women's Health* **2021**, *21*, 57. [CrossRef] [PubMed]
130. Cho, S.; Nam, A.; Kim, H.; Chay, D.; Park, K.; Cho, D.J.; Park, Y.; Lee, B. Clinical effects of the levonorgestrel-releasing intrauterine device in patients with adenomyosis. *Am. J. Obstet. Gynecol.* **2008**, *198*, 373.e1–373.e7. [CrossRef] [PubMed]
131. Health Quality Ontario Levonorgestrel-Releasing Intrauterine System (52 mg) for Idiopathic Heavy Menstrual Bleeding: A Health Technology Assessment. *Ont. Health Technol. Assess. Ser.* **2016**, *16*, 1–119.
132. Claessens, E.A.; Cowell, C.A. Acute adolescent menorrhagia. *Am. J. Obstet. Gynecol.* **1981**, *139*, 277–280. [CrossRef]
133. Kadir, R.A.; Economides, D.L.; Sabin, C.; Pollard, D.; Lee, C.A. Assessment of menstrual blood loss and gynaecological problems in patients with inherited bleeding disorders. *Haemophilia* **1999**, *5*, 40–48. [CrossRef] [PubMed]
134. Lee, C.A. Women and inherited bleeding disorders: Menstrual issues. *Semin. Hematol.* **1999**, *36*, 21–27.
135. Kingman, C.; Kadir, R.; Lee, C.; Economides, D. The use of levonorgestrel-releasing intrauterine system for treatment of menorrhagia in women with inherited bleeding disorders. *BJOG Int. J. Obstet. Gynaecol.* **2004**, *111*, 1425–1428. [CrossRef]
136. Pisoni, C.N.; Cuadrado, M.J.; Khamashta, M.A.; Hunt, B.J. Treatment of menorrhagia associated with oral anticoagulation: Efficacy and safety of the levonorgestrel releasing intrauterine device (Mirena coil). *Lupus* **2006**, *15*, 877–880. [CrossRef]
137. Kadir, R.A.; Chi, C. Levonorgestrel intrauterine system: Bleeding disorders and anticoagulant therapy. *Contraception* **2007**, *75*, S123–S129. [CrossRef]
138. Lukes, A.S.; Reardon, B.; Arepally, G. Use of the levonorgestrel-releasing intrauterine system in women with hemostatic disorders. *Fertil. Steril.* **2008**, *90*, 673–677. [CrossRef]
139. Chi, C.; Huq, F.Y.; Kadir, R.A. Levonorgestrel-releasing intrauterine system for the management of heavy menstrual bleeding in women with inherited bleeding disorders: Long-term follow-up. *Contraception* **2011**, *83*, 242–247. [CrossRef] [PubMed]
140. Rimmer, E.; Jamieson, M.A.; James, P. Malposition and expulsion of the levonorgestrel intrauterine system among women with inherited bleeding disorders. *Haemophilia* **2013**, *19*, 933–938. [CrossRef]
141. Lu, M.; Yang, X. Levonorgestrel-releasing intrauterine system for treatment of heavy menstrual bleeding in adolescents with Glanzmann's Thrombasthenia: Illustrated case series. *BMC Women's Health* **2018**, *18*, 45. [CrossRef] [PubMed]
142. Li, H.; Li, C.; Shi, X.; Xia, M. Heavy menstrual bleeding due to primary myelofibrosis in a woman: A case report. *Am. J. Transl. Res.* **2021**, *13*, 12016–12020.
143. Brull, E.P.; Fernandes, A.; Monteiro, I.; Bahamondes, L.; Juliato, C.R.T. Safety and bleeding patterns of the levonorgestrel 52-mg intrauterine system among women with thrombosis or coagulopathy. *Int. J. Gynecol. Obstet.* **2020**, *151*, 355–361. [CrossRef]
144. Campos, R.R.; Baêta, T.; Silva-Filho, A.; Rezende, S.M.; Rocha, A.L.L. Use of a levonorgestrel 52-mg intrauterine system in the control of abnormal uterine bleeding in women with inherited bleeding disorders. *Contraception* **2020**, *102*, 254–258. [CrossRef]
145. Brignardello-Petersen, R.; El Alayli, A.; Husainat, N.; Kalot, M.A.; Shahid, S.; Aljabirii, Y.; Britt, A.; Alturkmani, H.J.; El-Khechen, H.; Motaghi, S.; et al. Gynecologic and obstetric management of women with von Willebrand disease: Summary of 3 systematic reviews of the literature. *Blood Adv.* **2022**, *6*, 228–237. [CrossRef]
146. Luukkainen, T.; Nilsson, G.; Allonen, H.; Haukkamaa, M.; Toivenen, J. Intrauterine release of levonorgestrel. In *Long-Acting Contraception*; Papers Presented at the symposium on Long-Acting Contraception; Goldsmith, A., Toppozada, M., Eds.; Johnson-Lindroth, Inc.: Alexandria, Egypt; Chicago, IL, USA, 1983; pp. 167–173.
147. Lowe, R.F.; Prata, N. Hemoglobin and serum ferritin levels in women using copper-releasing or levonorgestrel-releasing intrauterine devices: A systematic review. *Contraception* **2013**, *87*, 486–496. [CrossRef] [PubMed]
148. Rana, M.; Saxena, P.; Firdous, N. Comparison of levonorgestrel and copper releasing intrauterine contraceptive device on body iron stores and menstrual bleeding patterns: Experience on Indian women. *Eur. Rev. Med. Pharmacol. Sci.* **2012**, *16*, 230–234. [PubMed]

149. Bahamondes, L.; Petta, C.A.; Fernandes, A.; Monteiro, I. Use of the levonorgestrel-releasing intrauterine system in women with endometriosis, chronic pelvic pain and dysmenorrhea. *Contraception* **2007**, *75*, S134–S139. [CrossRef]
150. Yucel, N.; Baskent, E.; Balci, B.K.; Goynumer, G. The levonorgestrel-releasing intrauterine system is associated with a reduction in dysmenorrhoea and dyspareunia, a decrease in CA 125 levels, and an increase in quality of life in women with suspected endometriosis. *Aust. N. Z. J. Obstet. Gynaecol.* **2018**, *58*, 560–563. [CrossRef] [PubMed]
151. Yoo, H.J.; Lee, M.A.; Ko, Y.B.; Yang, J.B.; Kang, B.H.; Lee, K.H. The efficacy of the levonorgestrel-releasing intrauterine system in perimenopausal women with menorrhagia or dysmenorrhea. *Arch. Gynecol. Obstet.* **2012**, *285*, 161–166. [CrossRef] [PubMed]
152. Lindh, I.; Milsom, I. The influence of intrauterine contraception on the prevalence and severity of dysmenorrhea: A longitudinal population study. *Hum. Reprod.* **2013**, *28*, 1953–1960. [CrossRef] [PubMed]
153. Kelekci, S.; Kelekci, K.H.; Yilmaz, B. Effects of levonorgestrel-releasing intrauterine system and T380A intrauterine copper device on dysmenorrhea and days of bleeding in women with and without adenomyosis. *Contraception* **2012**, *86*, 458–463. [CrossRef] [PubMed]
154. Sheng, J.; Zhang, W.Y.; Zhang, J.P.; Lu, D. The LNG-IUS study on adenomyosis: A 3-year follow-up study on the efficacy and side effects of the use of levonorgestrel intrauterine system for the treatment of dysmenorrhea associated with adenomyosis. *Contraception* **2009**, *79*, 189–193. [CrossRef] [PubMed]
155. Wildemeersch, D.; Schacht, E.; Wildemeersch, P. Treatment of primary and secondary dysmenorrhea with a novel 'frameless' intrauterine levonorgestrel-releasing drug delivery system: A pilot study. *Eur. J. Contracept. Reprod. Health Care* **2001**, *6*, 192–198. [CrossRef]
156. Gold, M.A.; Johnson, L.M. Intrauterine devices and adolescents. *Curr. Opin. Obstet. Gynecol.* **2008**, *20*, 464–469. [CrossRef]
157. Jatlaoui, T.C.; Riley, H.E.; Curtis, K.M. The safety of intrauterine devices among young women: A systematic review. *Contraception* **2017**, *95*, 17–39. [CrossRef]
158. Buhling, K.J.; Hauck, B.; Dermout, S.; Ardaens, K.; Marions, L. Understanding the barriers and myths limiting the use of intrauterine contraception in nulliparous women: Results of a survey of European/Canadian healthcare providers. *Eur. J. Obstet. Gynecol. Reprod. Biol.* **2014**, *183*, 146–154. [CrossRef] [PubMed]
159. Worl Health Organization. *Medical Eligibility Criteria for Contraceptive Use*; WHO: Geneva, Switzerland, 2015.
160. Hauck, B.; Costescu, D. Barriers and Misperceptions Limiting Widespread Use of Intrauterine Contraception Among Canadian Women. *J. Obstet. Gynaecol. Can.* **2015**, *37*, 606–616. [CrossRef]
161. Godfrey, E.M.; Memmel, L.M.; Neustadt, A.; Shah, M.; Nicosia, A.; Moorthie, M.; Gilliam, M. Intrauterine contraception for adolescents aged 14–18 years: A multicenter randomized pilot study of Levonorgestrel-releasing intrauterine system compared to the Copper T 380A. *Contraception* **2010**, *81*, 123–127. [CrossRef] [PubMed]
162. Aslam, N.; Blunt, S.; Latthe, P. Effectiveness and tolerability of levonorgestrel intrauterine system in adolescents. *J. Obstet. Gynaecol.* **2010**, *30*, 489–491. [CrossRef] [PubMed]
163. Bayer, L.L.; Hillard, P.J.A. Use of Levonorgestrel Intrauterine System for Medical Indications in Adolescents. *J. Adolesc. Health* **2013**, *52*, S54–S58. [CrossRef] [PubMed]
164. Adeyemi-Fowode, O.A.; Bercaw-Pratt, J.L. Intrauterine Devices: Effective Contraception with Noncontraceptive Benefits for Adolescents. *J. Pediatr. Adolesc. Gynecol.* **2019**, *32*, S2–S6. [CrossRef]
165. Beatty, M.N.; Blumenthal, P.D. The levonorgestrel-releasing intrauterine system: Safety, efficacy, and patient acceptability. *Ther. Clin. Risk Manag.* **2009**, *5*, 561–574. [CrossRef] [PubMed]
166. Bitzer, J.; Rapkin, A.; Soares, C.N. Managing the risks of mood symptoms with LNG-IUS: A clinical perspective. *Eur. J. Contracept. Reprod. Health Care* **2018**, *23*, 321–325. [CrossRef]
167. Jiménez, M.F.; Vetori, D.; Fagundes, P.A.; de Freitas, F.M.; Cunha-Filho, J.S. Subendometrial microvascularization and uterine artery blood flow in IUD-induced side effects (levonorgestrel intrauterine system and copper intrauterine device). *Contraception* **2008**, *78*, 324–327. [CrossRef]

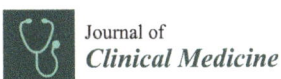

Review

Alternative Insertion Site of Nexplanon: Description of a Case Report and Systematic Review of the Literature

Guglielmo Stabile [1,*], Carmelina Foti [2], Denise Mordeglia [2], Davide De Santo [1], Francesco Paolo Mangino [1], Antonio Simone Laganà [3] and Giuseppe Ricci [1,2]

1. Institute for Maternal and Child Health, IRCCS Burlo Garofolo, 34100 Trieste, Italy; davide.desanto@burlo.trieste.it (D.D.S.); francesco.mangino@burlo.trieste.it (F.P.M.); giuseppe.ricci@burlo.trieste.it (G.R.)
2. Department of Medicine, Surgery and Health Sciences, University of Trieste, 34127 Trieste, Italy; carmelina.foti@burlo.trieste.it (C.F.); denise.mordeglia@burlo.trieste.it (D.M.)
3. Unit of Gynecologic Oncology, ARNAS "Civico—Di Cristina—Benfratelli", Department of Health Promotion, Mother and Child Care, Internal Medicine and Medical Specialties (PROMISE), University of Palermo, 90127 Palermo, Italy; antoniosimone.lagana@unipa.it
* Correspondence: guglielmost@gmail.com

Abstract: The etonogestrel (ENG) implant is among the most effective reversible contraceptives. It can be a good option for patients with different chronic diseases due to no clinically significant effects on lipid metabolism or liver function. Some limitations in the use of this type of device are represented by social and psychiatric disorders, where the easy accessibility of the device becomes a negative feature. In these patients several cases of self-removal or damage to the device have been reported. We report the successful insertion of the Nexplanon® device into the scapular region in a young woman with a chronic psychiatric disorder. To verify the presence in the literature of other possible implantation sites, we performed a systematic review of the literature on Pubmed, Google scholar and Scopus from 2000 to 2021 using different combinations of the following terms: (Nexplanon), (contraceptive implant), (insertion). Two manuscripts with three cases were detected. Nexplanon® was implanted in the upper back. In all cases, there were no complications during the insertions and the follow up demonstrated no side effects with contraceptive efficacy. Our report and review is a further confirmation that the scapular region can become a valid insertion site, maintaining good efficacy and safety of the subcutaneous device.

Keywords: Nexplanon; subcutaneous device; etonogestrel implant; alternative insertion; implantation site; contraceptive implant

1. Introduction

Nexplanon® is a progestin contraceptive implant placed under the skin on the inner side of the non-dominant upper arm for long-acting reversible contraception. It contains 68 mg of ENG implant that is slowly released for three years; it is not impacted by individual characteristics and genetic variants

The ENG implant is among the most effective reversible contraceptives available, with efficacy as good or better than the sterilization procedures, but without the risk of invasive surgery [1–3].

Implant contraceptives can be a good option for patients with chronic diseases because, beyond their need for highly effective contraception, there are no clinically significant effects on lipid metabolism or liver function. According to the criteria of eligibility of contraception [4,5], their use is contraindicated in women with serious conditions such as severe cirrhosis and other benign and malignant liver tumors, thromboembolic or ischemic heart disease, suspicious vaginal bleeding, breast cancer, systemic lupus erythematosus and anti-phospholipid positivity, or hypersensitivity to any component of the method [6].

Other possible limitations are represented by social and psychiatric disorders, where the easy accessibility of the device becomes a negative feature. In these patients, several cases of self-removal or damage (breaking or bending) of the device have been reported in the literature.

We report the successful insertion of the subcutaneous device in the scapular region in a young woman with chronic psychiatric disorder. To verify the presence in the literature of other possible implantation sites, we performed a systematic review of the literature on Pubmed, Google scholar and Scopus.

2. Case

A 16-year-old girl presented to our hospital, accompanied by her mother, for a menstrual disorder: she reported long periods of amenorrhea over the last years. The patient suffered from borderline personality disorder with marked affective instability and impulsivity with self-harm, which had caused multiple superficial cuts along the forearms bilaterally and on the right thigh. The patient was on chronic lithium therapy with poor control of psychiatric symptoms. Options were discussed and the mother, the legal administrator, refused the intrauterine device (IUD) because of the maidenhood status of the daughter, and the estrogen-progestogen pills due to the difficulty of ensuring daily intake. Additionally, the vaginal ring and transdermal contraceptive patch were inappropriate due to low adherence to treatment. For these reasons, the best option was the insertion of the subcutaneous device, Nexplanon®. Because of the patient's psychiatric illness, the typical site at arm level was not recommended due to the high risk of self-removal or damage.

The risks and benefits of the subcutaneous device were explained to the mother and the patient, underlining that in the literature there are very few cases of alternative insertion site. They gave the consent for Nexplanon® placement in a different unreachable body site.

After skin disinfection and local anesthesia, Nexplanon® was placed in the right scapular region without any complications (Figure 1).

At the follow-up visits (3 and 6 months after insertion), the patient reported normalization of the menstrual cycle without any side effects or discomfort related to the implant such as headaches, acne, pain, breast pain or depression. The implant remained superficial and palpable in the same position. However, she did not seem to pay attention to the implant and did not try to remove it.

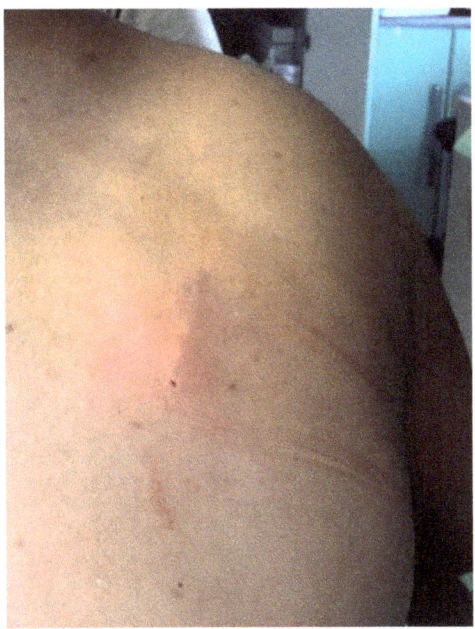

Figure 1. Nexplanon's insertion site.

3. Materials and Methods

This research was approved by our Institutional Review Board (RC 08/2020).

MEDLINE (PubMed), Google Scholar and Scopus databases were searched up to December 2021. The manuscripts considered were published from 2000 up to December 2021.

Only articles in English were included in the search. The research strategy adopted included different combinations of the following terms: (Nexplanon) AND (contraceptive implant) AND (insertion).

For the selection of the papers, we included articles that focused on cases of alternative sites of Nexplanon implantation. We examined in our review, the age and the history of patients, symptoms, the medical reason for a different Nexplanon® implant, the procedure and the follow up.

We excluded from the review studies with different topics like aberrations from procedure for insertion and removal, and case complications such as infections, migrations, embolism, lipoatrophy and adverse reactions.

All studies identified were examined for year, citation, title, authors, abstract and their full texts. Duplicates were identified through manual screening performed by one researcher and then removed. PRISMA guidelines were followed. The PRISMA flow diagram of the selection process is provided in Figure 2. The systematic review was not submitted to Prospero as only a limited number of case reports were found in the literature. For the eligibility process, three authors independently screened the title and abstracts of all non-duplicated papers and excluded those not pertinent to the topic (G.S., C.F., D.M.). The same three authors independently reviewed the full text of papers that passed the first screening and identified those to be included in the review. Discrepancies were resolved by consensus. Two manuscripts were detected through the references of the works that had been identified with the research on PubMed, Scopus and Google Scholar [7].

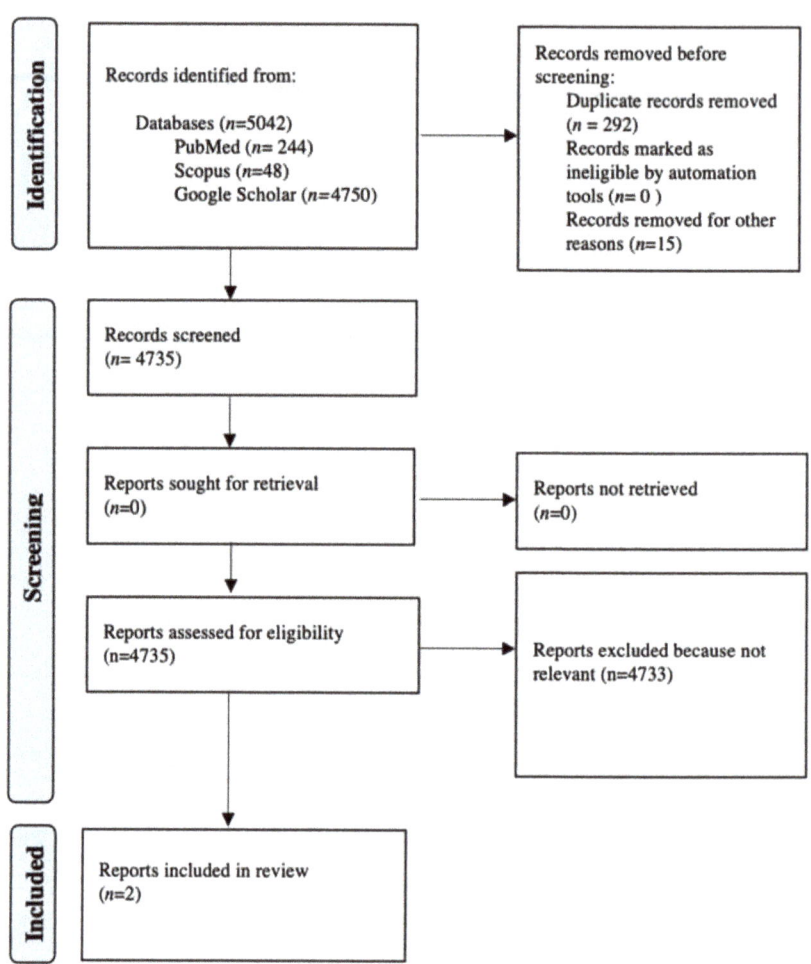

Figure 2. PRISMA flow diagram.

Because this contraceptive method is cutting edge, the studies included are all case reports. For this reason, we present the data in a descriptive manner.

4. Results

We identified, through database searching, 5042 records (n = 244 from MEDLINE; n = 48 from Scopus; n = 4750 from Google Scholar). We removed duplicates (n = 292) and others written in non-English (n = 15). After screening and exclusion of all records on different topics, two manuscripts were detected as eligible in our review (Table 1).

Table 1. Review of the literature.

Title	Authors	Age and Previous Pregnancies	Desease	Medical Reason of Nexplanon Different Insertion	Alternative Site	Anesthesia	Contraceptive Efficacy	Follow Up
Alternative insertion site in the scapular region for etonogestrel contraceptive implant (Nexplanon®) [8]	David Pragout MD, Francois Darrouzain Pharm.D PhD, Henri Marret MD PhD. "European Journal of Obstetrics & Gynecology and Reproductive Biology" 2018	23 years old nulliparous	Chronic psychotic illness that causes aggressive and self-harming behavior	Frequent self inflicted lacerations	Right lower scapular region	Local anesthesia	Good	3-6-18 months NO side effects, apart from amenorrhea
Novel location of Nexplanon® placement in developmentally delayed twins: a case report [9]	Maura Quinlan MD MPH, Melissa Matulich MD. "Journal of Pediatric and Adolescent Gynecology" 2018	14 years old nulliparous	Global developmental delay, premenstrual behavior changes, hygiene issues with menses	Habitually pick at their skin	Upper back, parallel and 3 cm lateral to the spinous process at the level of the axilla	One twin: general anesthesia other twin: local anesthesia after oral anxiolytic	Good	No cyclic behavior issues have been noted and spotting has been tolerable

They report three cases of young women (two twins and another girl) that suffer from chronic neurological diseases and psychotic symptoms, and that frequently self-inflict lacerations on their skin. For this reason, Nexplanon® was implanted in the upper back. Only one had it placed under general anesthesia. There were no complications during the insertions and the follow up demonstrated no side effects with a good compliance and contraceptive efficacy.

5. Discussion

The Nexplanon® implant is a 4 cm rod-shaped barium sulphate, containing 68 mg ENG.

Peak serum concentration (266 pg/mL) of ENG is achieved within 1 day after insertion, suppressing ovulation, which requires only 90 or more pg/mL [10]. Bioavailability of the ENG implant remains at nearly 100% over 2 years of use. After implant removal, serum ENG concentrations become undetectable within 1 week [11]. The contraceptive effect is obtained through two complementary mechanisms: the progestin inhibits the gonadotropin secretion and ovulation, and it causes changes in cervical mucus and tubal motility that are unfavorable to sperm migration [12].

To date, the common site of insertion is at the level of the medial face of the non-dominant arm with local anesthesia, 8 to 10 cm above the medial epicondyle of the non-dominant arm, 3–5 cm away from the sulcus between the biceps and triceps muscles that contains a large neurovascular bundle [13,14]. This anatomic area is easily accessible without important vessels and with low risk of device migration.

Complications are rare; they are reported in 0.3–1% of insertions and 0.2–1.75 of removals [15,16]. These include infection, hematoma formation, local irritation or rash, expulsion, and allergic reaction [17]. The implant may migrate a short distance (less than 2 cm) over time. There are two case reports of neurologic symptoms during ENG implant insertion in the literature: nerve injury to branches of the medial antebrachial cutaneous nerve during placement and neuropathy due to contact of the implant with the medial antebrachial cutaneous nerve [18,19]. In rare cases, intravascular insertion may cause migration of the implant to the pulmonary artery [20,21].

In the literature, there are very few cases of insertion in other regions (the median supraumbilical region and medial side of the thigh have been suggested) because of the presence of vulnerable nerves and vessels in the inner arm [8]. The scapular region is one of the less self-accessible areas and the anatomic site is distant from neurovascular structures, even in the case of accidental deep insertion, although it does not present a greater risk of migration.

We report the three cases described in the literature of insertion localized at the back and the results were good for compliance by the patient and contraceptive efficacy as demonstrated by the estrogen levels. In these cases, including the case from our institute, all patients shared similar diseases with psychiatric and neurological symptoms. In general, insertion of Nexplanon® in other sites could be a good possibility in patients with social problems (e.g., drug addiction) or with skin and neuromuscular diseases of the upper limbs.

The strength of our study is the novelty and the presentation of a very rare case (only three others present in the literature) and the long period of time reviewed in the literature: we analysed the cases of alternative sites of implantation of contraceptive device from over the last 21 years. All the studies selected during the eligibility phase were further evaluated by manual comparison of populations, study settings and authors to avoid overlapping cases.

The limitation of our study is the retrospective nature of it and the main risk of bias is represented by the presence of all case reports among the papers selected, due to the rarity of this complication.

6. Conclusions

There are a significant number of psychiatric and social conditions that would benefit from the possibility of having an effective and safe contraceptive device, not easily accessible by the user. It becomes imperative to think of an alternative insertion site in order to meet all the needs of patients. As demonstrated by the previous cases described in the literature, our case report is a further confirmation that the scapular region can become a valid insertion site, because this anatomical region does not reduce the efficacy and safety of the subcutaneous device and does not lead to an increased risk of complications. Unfortunately, we do not know what the removal of the device will look like. For this reason, it is necessary to carry out a study that can systematically test this anatomical region as a possible alternative insertion site, evaluating the insertion, removal and associated complications compared to the common site.

Author Contributions: Conceptualization, G.S., D.D.S., G.R. and D.M.; methodology, C.F.; software, C.F.; validation, G.R., A.S.L. and F.P.M.; formal analysis, G.S. and C.F.; investigation, C.F. and A.S.L.; resources, G.S.; data curation, C.F.; writing—original draft preparation, GS and C.F.; writing—review and editing, G.S. and F.P.M.; visualization, D.D.S. and G.R.; supervision, G.R.; project administration, G.S.; All authors have read and agreed to the published version of the manuscript.

Funding: This research received no external funding.

Institutional Review Board Statement: The study was conducted in accordance with the Declaration of Helsinki and approved by the Institutional Review Board of the IRCCS Burlo Garofolo (RC 08/2020).

Informed Consent Statement: Informed consent was obtained from all subjects involved in the study.

Data Availability Statement: All data were included in this manuscript.

Conflicts of Interest: The authors declare no conflict of interest.

References

1. Mansour, D.; Inki, P.; Gemzell-Danielsson, K. Efficacy of contraceptive methods: A review of the literature. *Eur. J. Contracept. Reprod. Health Care* **2010**, *15*, 4–16. [CrossRef] [PubMed]
2. Stabile, G.; Romano, F.; De Santo, D.; Sorrentino, F.; Nappi, L.; Cracco, F.; Ricci, G. Case Report: Bowel Occlusion Following the Use of Barbed Sutures in Abdominal Surgery. A Single-Center Experience and Literature Review. *Front Surg.* **2021**, *8*, 626505. [CrossRef]
3. Buzzaccarini, G.; Stabile, G.; Török, P.; Petousis, S.; Mikuš, M.; Della Corte, L.; Barra, F.; Laganà, A.S. Surgical Approach for Enlarged Uteri: Further Tailoring of vNOTES Hysterectomy. *J. Investig. Surg.* **2022**, *35*, 924–925. [CrossRef] [PubMed]
4. World Health Organization. Reproductive Health. In *Medical Eligibility Criteria for Contraceptive Use*; World Health Organization: Geneva, Switzerland, 2010.
5. Rocca, M.L.; Palumbo, A.R.; Visconti, F.; Di Carlo, C. Safety and Benefits of Contraceptives Implants: A Systematic Review. *Pharmaceuticals* **2021**, *14*, 548. [CrossRef] [PubMed]
6. Palomba, S.; Falbo, A.; Di Cello, A.; Materazzo, C.; Zullo, F. Nexplanon: The new implant for long-term contraception. A comprehensive descriptive review. *Gynecol. Endocrinol.* **2012**, *28*, 710–721. [CrossRef] [PubMed]
7. Stabile, G.; Mordeglia, D.; Romano, F.; Carlucci, S.; Mangino, F.P.; Nappi, L.; Sorrentino, F.; De Manzini, N.; Ricci, G. Postcoital Vaginal Perforation and Evisceration in Women with No Prior Pelvic Surgery: Laparoscopic Management and Systematic Review of the Literature. *Int. J. Environ. Res. Public Health* **2021**, *18*, 9746. [CrossRef] [PubMed]
8. Pragout, D.; Darrouzain, F.; Marret, H. Alternative insertion site in the scapular region for etonogestrel contraceptive implant (Nexplanon®). *Eur. J. Obs. Gynecol. Reprod. Biol.* **2018**, *224*, 207–208. [CrossRef] [PubMed]
9. Quinlan, M.; Matulich, M. Novel Location of Nexplanon Placement in Developmentally Delayed Twins: A Case Report. *J. Pediatric Adolesc. Gynecol.* **2018**, *31*, 169. [CrossRef]
10. Mäkäräinen, L.; van Beek, A.; Tuomivaara, L.; Asplund, B.; Coelingh Bennink, H. Ovarian function during the use of a single contraceptive implant: Implanon compared with Norplant. *Fertil. Steril.* **1998**, *69*, 714–721. [CrossRef]
11. Wenzl, R.; van Beek, A.; Schnabel, P.; Huber, J. Pharmacokinetics of etonogestrel released from the contraceptive implant Implanon. *Contracept.* **1998**, *58*, 283–288. [CrossRef]
12. Croxatto, H.B. Mechanisms that explain the contraceptive action of progestin implants for women. *Contraception* **2002**, *65*, 21–27. [CrossRef]
13. Walling, M.R. New insertion site for Nexplanon insertion. *BMJ Sex Reprod. Health* **2019**, *3*, bmjsrh-2018-200279. [CrossRef] [PubMed]
14. Available online: www.nexplanon.co.uk/training (accessed on 5 April 2022).
15. Gillies, R.; Scougall, P.; Nicklin, S. Etonogestrel implants—Case studies of median nerve injury following removal. *Aust. Fam. Physician* **2011**, *40*, 799–800. [PubMed]

16. Mascarenhas, L. Insertion and removal of Implanon: Practical considerations. *Eur. J. Contracept. Reprod. Health Care* **2000**, *2*, 29–34.
17. Available online: https://www.accessdata.fda.gov/drugsatfda_docs/label/2019/021529s018lbl.pdf (accessed on 5 April 2022).
18. Hindy, J.R.; Souaid, T.; Larus, C.T.; Glanville, J.; Aboujaoude, R. Nexplanon migration into a subsegmental branch of the pulmonary artery: A case report and review of the literature. *Medicine* **2020**, *99*, e18881. [CrossRef] [PubMed]
19. Barlow-Evans, R.; Jaffer, K.; Balogun, M. Migration of a Nexplanon contraceptive implant to the pulmonary artery. *BMJ Case Rep.* **2017**, *2017*, bcr2017219259. [CrossRef] [PubMed]
20. Wechselberger, G.; Wolfram, D.; Pülzl, P.; Soelder, E.; Schoeller, T. Nerve injury caused by removal of an implantable hormonal contraceptive. *Am. J. Obs. Gynecol.* **2006**, *195*, 323–326. [CrossRef] [PubMed]
21. O'Grady, E.E.; Power, D.M. Ulnar nerve injury on removal of a contraceptive implant. *Practitioner* **2016**, *260*, 21–24. [PubMed]

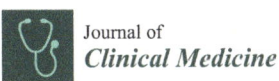

Journal of
Clinical Medicine

Review

Bleeding Patterns of Oral Contraceptives with a Cyclic Dosing Regimen: An Overview

David F. Archer [1], Diana Mansour [2] and Jean-Michel Foidart [3,4,*]

1. Department of Obstetrics and Gynecology, Clinical Research Center, Eastern Virginia Medical School, Norfolk, VA 23507, USA
2. Department of Sexual Health, New Croft Centre, Newcastle Hospitals, Community Health, Newcastle upon Tyne NE1 6ND, UK
3. Estetra SRL, Mithra Pharmaceuticals, 4000 Liège, Belgium
4. Department of Obstetrics and Gynecology, University of Liège, 4000 Liège, Belgium
* Correspondence: jfevaconsulting@gmail.com

Abstract: Bleeding irregularities are one of the major reasons for discontinuation of oral contraceptives (OCs), and therefore clinicians need to set expectations during consultations. In this review we provide an overview of bleeding data of recently marketed cyclic combined OCs (COCs) and one progestin-only pill (POP). We evaluated data from phase 3 trials (≥12 months) used to gain regulatory approval. Overall, each type of OC has its own specific bleeding pattern. These patterns however were assessed by using different bleeding definitions, which hampers comparisons between products. In COCs, the estrogen balances the effects of the progestin on the endometrium, resulting in a regular bleeding pattern. However, this balance seems lost if a too low dose of ethinylestradiol (EE) (e.g., 10 µg in EE/norethindrone acetate 1 mg) is used in an attempt to lower the risk of venous thromboembolism. Replacement of EE by 17β-estradiol (E2) or E2 valerate could lead to suboptimal bleeding profile due to destabilization of the endometrium. Replacement of EE with estetrol (E4) 15 mg in the combination with drospirenone (DRSP) 3 mg is associated with a predictable and regular scheduled bleeding profile, while the POP containing DRSP 4 mg in a 24/4 regimen is associated with a higher rate of unscheduled and absence of scheduled bleeding than combined products.

Keywords: oral contraceptives; bleeding pattern; ethinylestradiol; estetrol; estradiol; drospirenone; norethindrone acetate; nomegestrol acetate; dienogest

Citation: Archer, D.F.; Mansour, D.; Foidart, J.-M. Bleeding Patterns of Oral Contraceptives with a Cyclic Dosing Regimen: An Overview. *J. Clin. Med.* **2022**, *11*, 4634. https://doi.org/10.3390/jcm11154634

Academic Editors: Francesco Maria Primiero and Giuseppe Benagiano

Received: 20 June 2022
Accepted: 30 July 2022
Published: 8 August 2022

Publisher's Note: MDPI stays neutral with regard to jurisdictional claims in published maps and institutional affiliations.

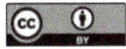

Copyright: © 2022 by the authors. Licensee MDPI, Basel, Switzerland. This article is an open access article distributed under the terms and conditions of the Creative Commons Attribution (CC BY) license (https://creativecommons.org/licenses/by/4.0/).

1. Introduction

Bleeding irregularities, including absence of scheduled bleeding (withdrawal bleeding), changes in volume of blood loss or duration of scheduled bleeding, and bleeding (including spotting) on unexpected days (unscheduled bleeding), are a well-known side effect of hormonal contraception. Such bleeding irregularities are often reported at the start of contraceptive use, especially by first time users, and diminish or disappear after the first three months [1,2]. However, it is one of the major reasons to discontinue oral contraceptives [1–3]. The occurrence of bleeding irregularities depends on the type of oral contraceptive (OC) [4] but may also result from a lack of treatment adherence, interactions with other drugs or intercurrent illness, such as vomiting and diarrhea. Moreover, smoking and a high body mass index (BMI) increase the likelihood of bleeding irregularities [5,6].

Hormonal contraceptives contain either estrogen plus progestin (combined oral contraceptives, COCs) or progestin only (progestin-only pills, POPs). While progestins are primarily responsible for the contraceptive effect, the estrogenic component of a COC balances the effects of the progestin on the endometrium, resulting in a regular bleeding pattern. Currently, the majority of COCs contain the synthetic estrogen ethinylestradiol (EE). Over the years, EE has been reduced to doses as low as 10 µg in order to lower the risk of venous thromboembolism (VTE). Novel COCs have been introduced, replacing EE with

17β-estradiol (E2), its esterified prodrug E2 valerate (E2V), or by the fetal estrogen estetrol (E4), in an attempt to reduce the cardiovascular risk. For users of E2-containing COCs, the VTE risk appears slightly lower compared to levonorgestrel/EE-containing products [7,8]. For the E4-containing COC, real life data on VTE risk are not yet available, but the effects on hemostasis parameters are minimal [9].

Changes in the estrogen component of a COC, may change the stabilizing estrogenic effect on the endometrium and may consequently affect the bleeding pattern. In 2007, Bachmann and Korner [10] reviewed the bleeding patterns of OCs in clinical trials published between 1986 and 2006. They highlighted the need to use standardized reporting of bleeding patterns. Up to then, different methods were used in clinical research to analyze the bleeding patterns associated with hormonal contraceptive use. In 1986, the World Health Organization (WHO) published a standard with recommendations on collection and analysis of bleeding data based on a 90-day reference period, also referred to as the Belsey criteria [11]. The 90-day reference period defined in this standard does not distinguish between scheduled and unscheduled bleeding, which is one of the main reasons why these criteria were not uniformly applied [12]. In 2007, a new set of recommendations for standardization of data collection, study design, and analysis of bleeding data was published by Mishell et al. [13], with new definitions for bleeding parameters, including definitions for unscheduled and scheduled bleeding (Table 1).

Since the publication of Mishell et al. [13], new OCs have entered the market. In this review, we provide an overview of the bleeding data for recently marketed cyclic OCs.

Table 1. Terminology and definitions according to Mishell et al. [13].

Bleeding	Evidence of blood loss that requires the use of sanitary protection with a tampon, pad, or pantyliner.
Spotting	Evidence of minimal blood loss that does not require new use of any type of sanitary protection, including pantyliners.
Episode of bleeding	Bleeding and/or spotting days bounded on either end by 2 days of no bleeding or spotting.
Scheduled bleeding and withdrawal bleeding *	Any bleeding or spotting that occurs during hormone-free intervals regardless of the duration of the regimen and may continue into the first 4 days (Days 1–4) of the subsequent cycle of combined hormonal contraceptive (CHC) therapy.
Unscheduled bleeding #	Any bleeding that occurs while taking active hormones, regardless of the duration of regimen. Two exceptions: • Bleeding that begins during a hormone-free interval and continues through Days 1–4 of the subsequent active cycle should not be considered unscheduled. • Bleeding reported during Days 1–7 of the first cycle of any study medication should not be considered unscheduled.
Unscheduled spotting #	Any spotting that occurs while taking active hormones, regardless of the duration of regimen. Two exceptions: • Spotting that begins during a hormone-free interval and continues through Days 1–4 of the subsequent active cycle should not be considered unscheduled. • Spotting reported during Days 1–7 of the first cycle of any study medication should not be considered unscheduled.
Amenorrhea	Use of the term amenorrhea should be abandoned in the context of CHC therapy and replaced with absence of all bleeding and spotting.

* The use of traditional terminology (periods or menses) should be abandoned with regard to CHCs and replaced by the use of scheduled bleeding or withdrawal bleeding. Scheduled bleeding emphasizes to the woman that her bleeding with hormonal methods is not the same as menstruation. # Unscheduled means bleeding or spotting is not expected. The terms breakthrough bleeding and breakthrough spotting should be abandoned and replaced by unscheduled bleeding and unscheduled spotting.

2. Methods

We present an overview of bleeding data from phase 3 clinical trials with four cyclic COCs: estradiol valerate 1–3 mg/dienogest 2–3 mg (E2V/DNG Bayer Healthcare Pharmaceuticals, Wayne, NJ, USA), EE 10 µg/norethindrone acetate 1 mg (EE/NETA Abbvie, Chicago IL, USA), estradiol 1.5 mg/nomegestrol acetate 2.5 mg (E2/NOMAC Theramex Paris, France), and estetrol 15 mg /drospirenone 3 mg (E4/DRSP; Estetra SRL, Liège, Belgium), and of one cyclic POP: 4 mg DRSP-only (Exeltis Healthcare Madrid, Spain). The phase 3 trials with E2/NOMAC included the internal comparator drospirenone 3 mg/EE 30 µg (EE/DRSP), in a 21/7 treatment regimen (Tables 2 and 3). Tables 2 and 3 and Figure 1 also include data from a phase 3 trial with DRSP/EE in a 24/4 treatment regimen, as a historical reference for a 24/4 regimen, and the data of a phase 2 trial with E4/DRSP that included E2V/DNG as an internal comparator.

For the overview, we collected bleeding data from phase 3 contraceptive trials (with a duration of at least 12 months) that were used to gain regulatory approval. From public assessment reports of regulatory agencies, we gathered data on the incidence of scheduled and unscheduled bleeding per treatment cycle and on the number of bleeding days by reference period. Public assessment reports may contain more complete and correct data, as publications can come out before approval of the product in which final corrections are not yet incorporated. For this reason, the use of these data can add to the quality of reviews [14]. Based on a search of the FDA/EMA and the Australian regulatory Therapeutic Goods Administration database, we could retrieve the assessment reports of all five cyclic oral contraceptives. In addition to the reports from regulatory agencies, we used data from scientific publications on the individual or pooled phase 3 clinical trials. For this, we performed targeted searches in PubMed to find any peer-reviewed clinical articles published between July 2006 and April 2022 that were related to the phase 3 contraceptives trials used to gain regulatory approval. The following search terms were used: oral contraception, oral contraceptive, bleeding, bleeding pattern, phase 3, drospirenone, nomegestrol, dienogest, norethindrone acetate, ethinylestradiol, estradiol, estradiol valerate, and estetrol. As search terms such as "phase 3" and "bleeding" were not always used as keywords for the phase 3 clinical trials that were used for registration, we did not perform a systematic search, but emphasis was placed on articles that could add useful clinical information regarding the bleeding profile in these phase 3 contraceptive trials. In addition, any literature references mentioned in clinicaltrials.gov register [15] related to these phase 3 clinical trials were assessed. We found 13 publications on the phase 3 clinical trials that provided detailed information on the bleeding profile and included those in this overview. Table 2 provides an overview of the trials and sources (public assessment reports and scientific publications) used in this review.

Table 2. Clinical trials and pooled analyses used for presentation of the bleeding profiles.

Product/Brand Name	Treatment Regimen	Trial Identifier	Trial/Countries	Trial Start-Completion	No. Subjects/Age (Years)/BMI (kg/m²) *	Data Sources	Discontinuation Rate (%) Overall/Due to AEs/Due to Bleeding Related AEs
E2V/DNG Qlaira®/Natazia®	2/22/2/2	NCT00206583	Phase 3 US/CAN	March 2005–July 2007	490/18-35/≤30	Nelson 2014 [16] FDA assessment report [17]	35.1/13.9/5.1
		NCT00185289	Phase 3 EU	April 2004–July 2006	1377/18-50/≤30	Palacios 2010 [18] FDA assessment report [17]	21.4/10.2/2.5
		NCT01221831	Phase 2 Finland (6 cycles)	September 2010–September 2011	78/18-35/18-30	Apter 2016 [19]	10.3/NR/NR
EE/NETA 10 μg Lo Loestrin®	24/2/2	NCT00391807	Phase 3 US	November 2006–September 2008	1660/18-45/≤35	Archer 2013 [20] FDA assessment report [21]	41.7/10.7/3.8
E2/NOMAC Zoely®	24/4	NCT00511199	Phase 3 EU/Asia/AUS	May 2006–April 2008	1591/18-50/17-35	Mansour 2011 [22] AUSPAR [23]	28.2/18.2/4.0
		NCT00413062	Phase 3 US/LA/CAN	June 2006–July 2008	1666/18-50/17-35	Westhoff 2012 [24] AUSPAR [23]	40.7/17.3/3.8
		NCT00511199 NCT00413062	Pooled analysis	-	3233/18-50/17-35	Mansour 2017 [25]	34.7/17.9/3.9
E4/DRSP Nextstellis®/Drovelis®/Lydisilka®	24/4	NCT02817828	Phase 3 EU/RUS	June 2016–April 2018	1553/18-50/≤35	Gemzell Danielsson 2022 [26] FDA assessment report [27]	21.6/10.1/3.4
		NCT02817841	Phase 3 US/CAN	August 2016–November 2018	1864/16-50/≤35	Creinin 2021 [28] FDA assessment report [27]	45.5/9.7/2.7
		NCT01221831	Phase 2 Finland (6 cycles)	September 2010–September 2011	79/18-35/18-30	Apter 2016 [19]	8.9/NR/NR

Table 2. Cont.

Product/Brand Name	Treatment Regimen	Trial Identifier	Trial/Countries	Trial Start-Completion	No. Subjects/Age (Years)/BMI (kg/m²) *	Data Sources	Discontinuation Rate (%) Overall/Due to AEs/Due to Bleeding Related AEs
DRSP-only Slynd®/Slinda®	24/4	2010-021787-15	Phase 3 Europe	July 2011–March 2013	713/18–45/-	Archer 2015 [29] FDA assessment report [30]	27.8/12.3/4.2
		2011-002396-42	Phase 3 Europe (9 cycles)	August 2012–January 2014	858/18–45/-	Palacios 2020 [31] FDA assessment report [30]	19.8/9.6/3.3
		NCT02269241	Phase 3 US	October 2014–October 2017	1006/≥15/-	FDA assessment report [30] Kimble 2020 [32]	65.0/11.2/NR
		EudraCT 2010-021787-15 EudraCT 2011-002396-42 NCT02269241 EudraCT 2013-002300-13	Pooled analysis	-	2598/≥15/-	FDA assessment report [30]	39.5/10.9/NR
EE 30 µg/DRSP Yasmin®	21/7	NCT00511199	Phase 3 EU/Asia/AUS	May 2006–April 2008	535/18–50/17–35	Mansour 2011 [22] AUSPAR [33]	23.4/10.5/C.7
		NCT00413062	Phase 3 US/LA/CAN	June 2006–July 2008	554/18–50/17–35	Westhoff 2012 [24] AUSPAR [33]	37.9/10.1/1.8
		NCT00511199 NCT00413062	Pooled analysis	-	1084/18–50/17–35	Mansour 2017 [25]	30.9/10.3/1.3
EE 20 µg/DRSP Yaz®	24/4	Protocol 303740	Phase 3 US/EU/LA		1027/17–36/≤35	FDA assessment report [34] Bachman 2004 [35]	28.9/7.5/NR

AE, adverse event; AUSPAR, Australian Public Assessment Report for prescription medicines; BMI, body mass index; DRSP, drospirenone; DNG, dienogest; EE, ethinylestradiol; E2: 17β-estradiol; E2V, E2 valerate; E4, estetrol; FDA, Food and Drug Administration; NETA, norethindrone acetate; No, number; NOMAC, nomegestrol acetate; NR, not reported. * Criteria on age and BMI as provided by the investigators.

3. Results—Overview of Bleeding Patterns of Most Recently Marketed Cyclic OCs

All phase 3 clinical trials described here, except those with E4/DRSP and DRSP-only, started before publication of the Mishell definitions [13]. This implies that different methods were used for the collection methods, the definition of bleeding, and the type of analyses performed across the slected clinical trials. For all products, an expected bleeding period is defined, and bleeding outside this period is considered to be unscheduled bleeding, but the exact definitions of the characteristics of these periods are quite different (Table 3). Furthermore, the definitions used for bleeding and spotting were also different. In some trials, the use of panty liners was considered as bleeding (E4/DRSP and DRSP-only) while in the other trials the use of panty liners was considered as spotting (Table 3).

The term bleeding was often used for the combination of all bleeding events, including spotting, considering that spotting is a mild form of bleeding. Overall, this observed difference in methods for the assessment of bleeding across the different oral contraceptives means that comparisons between products should not be made, with the exception of when two products are used in the same trial.

Figure 1 presents the incidence of scheduled bleeding, unscheduled bleeding, and absence of scheduled bleeding by cycle for each of the different OCs displayed above each subfigure. Although unscheduled bleeding data for Cycle 1 are included in the figure, it should be noted that this cycle is not evaluable for unscheduled bleeding, as in some instances, unscheduled bleeding is expected, especially in starters who initiate treatment on their first day of menstruation.

Table 3. Heterogeneity of bleeding/spotting data collection and definition in the phase 3 trials of the different OCs evaluated.

Product/Brand Name	Trial Identifier(s)	Data Collection	Definition of Spotting	Definition of Bleeding	Definition of Scheduled Bleeding
E2V/DNG Qlaira®/Natazia®	NCT0206583 NCT00185289	Paper diary	Vaginal blood in an amount that did not require the use of sanitary protection other than panty liner(s)	Vaginal bleeding the subject categorized as light, normal, or heavy, that, based on her personal experience, required the use of sanitary protection	Start at day 21 and continued without interruption. If no bleeding occurred until Cycle Day 20 of the next cycle, it was assessed as absence of scheduled bleeding in the previous treatment cycle.
EE/NETA 10 μg Lo Loestrin®	NCT00391807		Light bleeding not requiring sanitary protection (other than panty liners) was classified as spotting	Only spotting defined. All vaginal bleeding was recorded, including use of sanitary protection (other than panty liners)	First bleeding episode starting 4 days before the last day of active drug intake during a treatment cycle and 3 days after beginning treatment in the next treatment cycle.
E2/NOMAC Zoely®	NCT00511199 NCT00413062	Electronic diary	Vaginal bleeding requiring none or at most one pad/tampon per day	Vaginal bleeding requiring more than one pad/tampon per day	Within expected bleeding period (Day 25–Day 3 next cycle) including early and continued bleeding *.
E4/DRSP Nextstellis®/Drovelis®/Lydisilka®	NCT02817828 NCT02817841	Paper diary	Minimal vaginal blood loss that did not require the new use of sanitary protection, including panty liners	Vaginal blood loss that required the use of sanitary protection with a tampon, pad or panty liner	Within expected bleeding period (Day 25–Day 3 next cycle) including early and continued bleeding *.
DRSP only Slynd®/Slinda®	EudraCT 2010-021787-15 EudraCT 2011-002396-42 NCT02269241	Electronic diary	Blood loss that did not require new use of any type of sanitary protection	Blood loss that required the use of sanitary protection	Any bleeding or spotting that occurred during hormone-free intervals (defined as days 25–28 ± 1). Up to eight consecutive bleeding days were considered as scheduled bleeding days.
EE 30 μg/DRSP Yasmin®	NCT00511199 NCT00413062	Electronic diary	Vaginal bleeding requiring none or at most one pad/tampon per day	Vaginal bleeding requiring more than one pad/tampon per day	Within expected bleeding period (Day 21–Day 28 next cycle) including early and continued bleeding *.
EE 20 μg/DRSP Yaz® 24/4 regimen	Protocol 303740	Paper diary	No requirement for sanitary protection except panty liners	Need for sanitary protection	First bleeding after hormone withdrawal (i.e., day 25).

* Early bleeding started before Day 24 and continued in the expected bleeding period. Continued bleeding started in the expected bleeding period and continued thereafter. DRSP, drospirenone; DNG, dienogest; EE, ethinylestradiol; E2, 17β-estradiol; E2V, E2 valerate; E4, estetrol; FDA, Food and Drug Administration; NETA, norethindrone acetate; NOMAC, nomegestrol acetate.

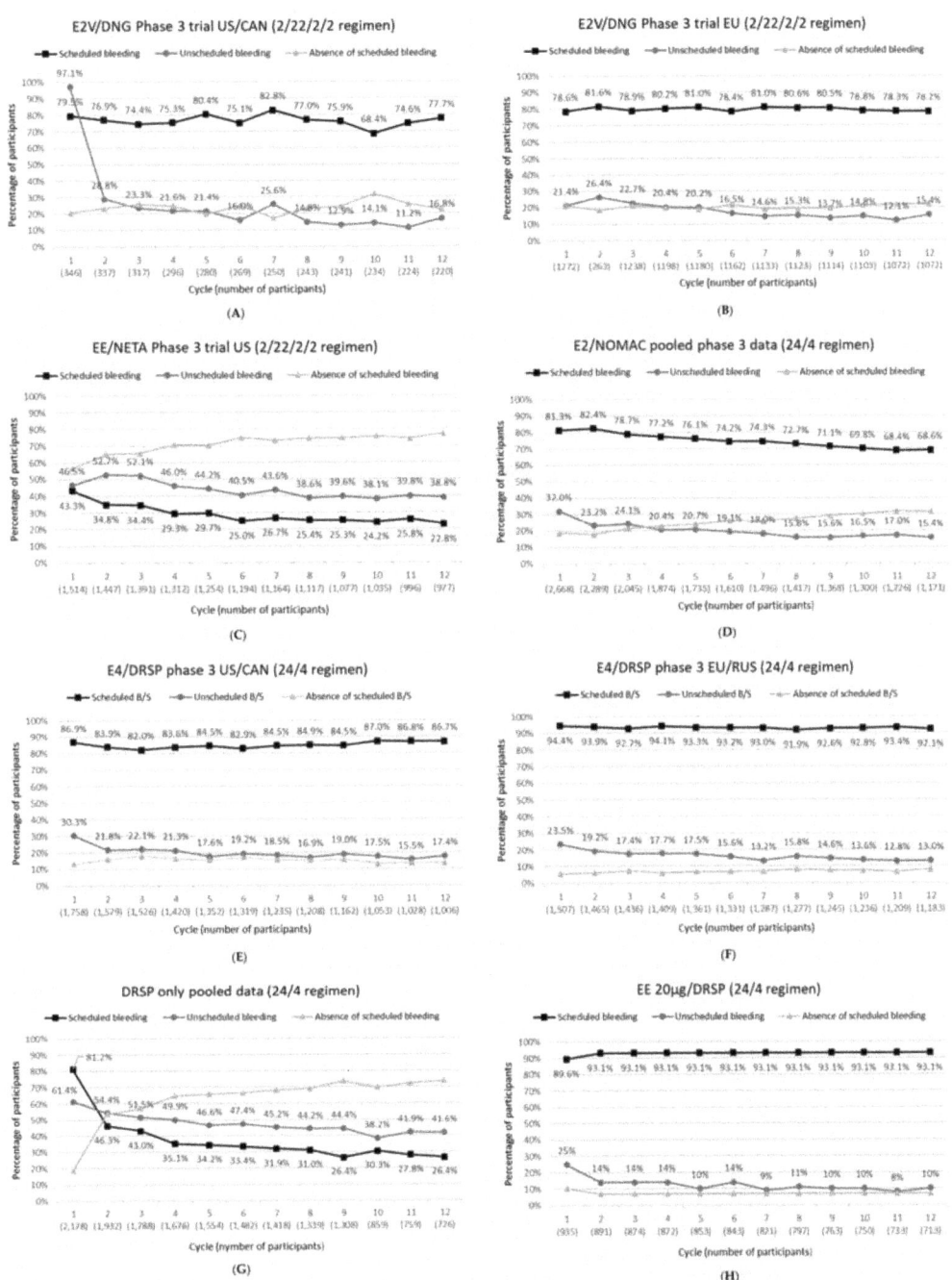

Figure 1. (A–H): Incidence of scheduled bleeding, unscheduled bleeding and absence of scheduled bleeding for each OC listed above each subfigure as a function of cycles.

Footnote for Figure 1: Data included: E2V/DNG trials NCT00206583 and NCT00185289; EE/NETA trial NCT00391807; E2/NOMAC pooled data of trials NCT00511199l and

NCT00511199; E4/DRSP trials NCT02817828 and NCT02817841; DRSP only: pooled data trials EudraCT 2010-021787-15, EudraCT 2011-002396-42, NCT02269241 and EudraCT 2013-002300-13; EE 20 µg/DRSP trial 303740.

Meaning of abbreviations: DRSP, drospirenone; DNG, dienogest; EE, ethinylestradiol; E2: 17β-estradiol; E2V, E2 valerate; E4, estetrol; FDA, Food and Drug Administration; NETA, norethindrone acetate; NOMAC, nomegestrol acetate.

3.1. E2V/DNG

E2V/DNG is the first combined oral contraceptive containing esterified estradiol, which is globally registered (first approval 2008). In contrast to other OCs discussed in this manuscript, E2V/DNG is a multiphasic pill containing varying dosages of the progestin and estrogen component. Treatment cycles start with 2 days of E2V 3 mg, followed by 5 days of DNG 2 mg/E2V 2 mg, 17 days of DNG 3 mg/E2V 2 mg, 2 days of E2V 1 mg and 2 days of inactive treatment, referred to as a 2/22/2/2-day treatment regimen.

During use of E2V/DNG, scheduled bleeding was stable throughout the trial period and occurred on average over cycles 1 to 12 in 76.5% of participants in the North American trial [16] and in 79.7% of participants in the European trial [17] (absence of scheduled bleeding 23.5% and 20.3%, respectively) (Figure 1A,B). The incidence of unscheduled bleeding diminished from 28.8% in Cycle 2 to 11.2% in Cycle 11 for the North American trial [16] and from 26.4% in Cycle 2 to 12.1% in Cycle 11 in the European trial [17] (Figure 1A,B). Discontinuation rates due to bleeding-related adverse events were 2.5% in the EU trial [18] and 5.1% in the US trial [16].

In addition to the two phase 3 trials, information on the bleeding profile of E2V/DNG is provided in a 7-month comparative trial with a COC containing levonorgestrel 100 µg and EE 20 µg (LNG/EE) in a 21/7 regimen [36]. The results of this trial showed that E2V/DNG has a lower rate of scheduled bleeding (77.7% to 83.2%) compared to LNG/EE (89.5% to 93.8%) ($p < 0.001$ per cycle), which may be related to the difference in treatment regimen. The incidence of unscheduled bleeding was similar for E2V/DNG (ranging between 10.5% and 18.6%) and LNG/EE (ranging between 9.9% and 17.1%).

3.2. EE/NETA

EE/NETA is a COC that combines NETA 1 mg with an ultra-low dose (10 µg) of the synthetic estrogen EE in a 24/2/2-day treatment regimen. The treatment cycle of EE/NETA starts with 24 days of NETA 1 mg/EE 10 µg, followed by 2 days of EE 10 µg and 2 days of ferrous fumarate 75 mg. EE/NETA is registered in the US (approval 2010).

Use of EE/NETA resulted in a low incidence of scheduled bleeding, which decreased from 43.3% in Cycle 1 to 22.8% in Cycle 12 (Figure 1C). Absence of scheduled bleeding was reported more frequently by switchers compared to new users and by older ($\geq$36 years) compared to younger participants [20]. Unscheduled bleeding occurred in 52.7% of participants in Cycle 2 and decreased to 38.8% in Cycle 12 (Figure 1C). Unscheduled bleeding tended to be higher in new users compared to switchers [20]. The percentage of participants discontinuing treatment due to bleeding-related adverse events was 3.8% [21].

3.3. E2/NOMAC

E2/NOMAC is a COC with a 24/4-day treatment regimen, with 24 tablets containing NOMAC 2.5 mg combined with E2 1.5 mg followed by 4 inactive tablets. E2/NOMAC is registered in Europe (approval 2011).

In the pooled phase 3 analysis, scheduled bleeding was reported by 82.4% of participants in Cycle 2, decreasing to 68.6% in Cycle 12 (Figure 1D), which was significantly lower compared to the reference COC EE/DRSP (ranging between 96.6% and 94.2%), an effect that may be related to the difference in treatment regimens (24/4 vs. 21/7) [23]. Absence of scheduled bleeding with E2/NOMAC was more common in participants aged $\geq$ 35 years (odds ratio [OR] 1.36, participants with a BMI $\geq$ 25 kg/m^2 (OR 1.47), switchers (OR 1.43), and smokers (OR 1.25 [25]. Unscheduled bleeding incidence ranged from 15.4 to 24.1%

over cycles 2 to 12 [23,25] (Figure 1D) and was significantly higher with E2/NOMAC compared to EE/DRSP [25]. Unscheduled bleeding appeared to be more common in starters (OR 1.38) and discontinuers (OR 1.19), but showed little association with age, BMI, and smoking [25]. During the phase 3 trials, 3.9% of participants discontinued E2/NOMAC use due to bleeding-related adverse events [25].

3.4. E4/DRSP

E4/DRSP is a COC containing E4, an estrogen produced in the human fetal liver [37] and manufactured for clinical use from a plant source [38–40]. E4/DRSP has a 24/4-day treatment regimen, with 24 tablets containing DRSP 3 mg combined with E4 15 mg (as monohydrate) followed by 4 inactive pills. E4/DRSP is globally registered (first approval 2021) [39,40].

During use of E4/DRSP in the phase 3 trials, the occurrence of scheduled bleeding was stable throughout the 12-month treatment period, with a regular scheduled bleeding in more than 92% of participants in the EU/RUS trial [26] and more than 83% of participants in the US/CAN trial [28] (Figure 1E,F). The percentage of women that reported unscheduled bleeding/spotting during treatment decreased from 19.2% in Cycle 2 to 13–18% from Cycle 3 onwards in the EU/RUS trial and from 21.8% in Cycle 2 to 15–20% from Cycle 5 onwards in the US/CAN trial (Figure 1E,F). The majority of unscheduled bleeding events were qualified by participants as spotting (not needing sanitary protection). The percentage of women that discontinued treatment due to bleeding problems was 3.4% in the EU/RUS trial and 2.7% in the US/CAN trial [26,28].

In addition to the phase 3 trials, a 6-cycle dose-finding phase 2 trial provided information on the bleeding pattern of E4/DRSP in comparison to E2V/DNG, which also contains a natural estrogen [19]. Results of this trial showed that the frequencies of unscheduled bleeding and absence of bleeding at Cycle 6 were lower with E4/DRSP (33.8% and 3.5%, respectively) compared to E2V/DNG (47.8% and 27.1%, respectively) at the end of treatment, suggesting a favorable bleeding pattern of E4/DRSP. Overall, E4/DRSP use resulted in a predictable bleeding pattern with limited unscheduled bleeding episodes, mostly defined as spotting.

3.5. DRSP-Only

In contrast to other available POPs that are provided as a continuous treatment, DRSP-only has a 24/4-day treatment regimen, consisting of 24 days of treatment with DRSP 4 mg, followed by 4 days of treatment with inactive tablets. The 24/4-day regimen DRSP-only was designed to reduce unscheduled bleeding, as this is a major reason for discontinuing the use of POPs. DRSP-only is globally registered (first approval 2019).

In the pooled phase 3 bleeding analysis, scheduled bleeding decreased from 81.2% in Cycle 1 and 46.3% in Cycle 2 to 26.4% in Cycle 12, while unscheduled bleeding decreased from 54.4% in Cycle 2 to 41.6% in Cycle 12 (Figure 1G). The number of participants discontinued due to bleeding irregularities was not provided for the pooled analysis but was reported to be 4.2% in the European trial [29].

The bleeding profile of the cyclic DRSP-only was compared with a typical continuous use of DSG-containing POP [31]. In this 9-cycle comparative phase 3 trial DRSP-only showed less bleeding compared to DSG. The rate of discontinuation due to bleeding-related adverse events was lower with DRSP-only (3.3%) compared to DSG (6.6%).

4. Discussion

In this review, we presented an overview of bleeding patterns of four cyclic COCs and the only cyclic POP marketed since 2008. We used data from public assessment reports of regulatory agencies, supplemented with data from scientific publications. In our literature search, we found that key words for bleeding, bleeding pattern, and phase 3 clinical trials were not uniformly applied, making it difficult to perform a systematic review. Instead, we chose to perform targeted searches for literature on bleeding reported during the phase 3 clinical trials of the five oral contraceptive products discussed in this review.

Overall, the more recent OCs each have their own specific bleeding pattern. It should be emphasized that based on presented data, a comparison of the different OCs cannot be made due to different definitions used in the trials. We therefore emphasize the importance to use uniform definitions for bleeding, spotting, and scheduled and unscheduled bleeding. For a detailed description of cycle control, separate reporting of bleeding and spotting episodes is recommended along with the consistent calculation of the bleeding duration, excluding users without any bleeding episodes. New recommendations on the standardization of bleeding data analysis has been published [41].

Three out of the four COCs contain a natural estrogenic component; E2V (E2V/DNG), E2 (E2/NOMAC), or E4 (E4/DRSP); the fourth COC contains an ultra-low dose of synthetic EE (EE/NETA 10 µg). The ultra-low dose of EE in EE/NETA is geared toward a safer product in an attempt to lower the risk of VTE. However, lowering the dose of EE (below 20 µg) leads to a reduced estrogenic effect on the endometrium, and a less favorable bleeding profile [42]. This is clearly reflected by the relatively high incidence of unscheduled bleeding and absence of scheduled bleeding in phase 3 trials with EE/NETA. Replacement of EE by E2 results in a suboptimal bleeding pattern due to destabilization of the endometrium. Users of E2/NOMAC experience unscheduled bleeding and absence of scheduled bleeding, although to a lesser extent compared to EE/NETA. In phase 3 trials, the use of E2V/DNG resulted in a more stable bleeding pattern, with a relatively high incidence of scheduled bleeding. This high incidence is probably ameliorated by the chosen definition of scheduled bleeding. For E2V/DNG, a scheduled bleeding episode was indeed defined as the first bleeding that started not earlier than Day 21 (i.e., not more than 4 days before DNG withdrawal) and continued without interruption. No end day of the bleeding period was defined. If no bleeding occurred until Day 20 of the next cycle, it was assessed as absence of scheduled bleeding in the previous treatment cycle. Otherwise, any bleeding occurring during the first 20 days of the next cycle caused the previous cycle to be considered as a cycle with scheduled bleeding. The rather unique definition of scheduled bleeding in studies with E2V/DNG evidently increases the proportion of scheduled bleeding episodes and makes a comparison with other OCs using Mishell's criteria impossible. In phase 3 trials, the use of E4/DRSP resulted in a predictable bleeding profile with a regular scheduled bleeding. The cyclic DRSP-only POP lacks estrogenic activity, and in phase 3 trials, using similar evaluation criteria as E4/DRSP, this resulted in a relatively high rate of unscheduled bleeding and absence of scheduled bleeding. In general, however, comparisons can be hampered by the use of different bleeding definitions, making comparisons between products impossible.

Older COCs have a 21/7-day treatment regimen, with doses of EE 30 µg, generally resulting in a regular bleeding profile with a consistent scheduled bleeding during the 7 hormone-free days, as is observed with EE 30µg/DRSP (scheduled bleeding > 90%). The more recent products have a 24/4-day regimen, with only 4 hormone-free days. This affects the bleeding profile, especially with respect to the occurrence of scheduled bleeding. Products containing a progestin with a longer half-life, such as DRSP ($t_{1/2}$ ~ 30 h [43]) and NOMAC ($t_{1/2}$ ~ 46 h [44]), may result in a delay of scheduled bleeding until the first day(s) of active tablet intake of the next cycle, because the progestin levels remain high during the first hormone-free days. It is important to note that from the user's perspective, the timing of the scheduled bleeding relative to tablet intake may not be an issue, as long as it is predictable and of acceptable length, but users should be informed about this possible delayed start of the withdrawal bleeding coinciding with the start of the next treatment cycle.

With EE/NETA and E2/NOMAC, the incidence of scheduled bleeding decreases over time, and at Cycle 12, only ~20% of participants using EE/NETA and ~70% of participants using E2/NOMAC experienced a scheduled bleeding. For E2V/DNG and E4/DRSP, the frequency of scheduled bleeding is consistent over time and appears lower with E2V/DNG

(~80%) compared to E4/DRSP (~90%). While a withdrawal bleeding during OC use does not represent physiological menstruation or serve a medical need, a regular monthly bleeding may be desirable, as it reassures the user that she is not pregnant [45,46]. Women considering the use of an OC with a low frequency of scheduled bleeding should be counseled appropriately.

Nowadays, many types of contraception are available, which makes counselling of potential users on the possibilities, the risks, and the potential benefits an important factor in the prescription of contraceptives. Because bleeding irregularities are one of the major reasons for discontinuation, potential users should receive adequate information on the expected bleeding pattern and the risk of bleeding irregularities. The newer OCs presented here each have their own particular bleeding pattern. Data in this review may provide prescribers with useful information on the bleeding pattern of these OCs needed for counselling of potential users.

Author Contributions: All authors (D.F.A., D.M. and J.-M.F.) have substantially contributed to the work. All authors have read and agreed to the published version of the manuscript.

Funding: Authors received no funding for the preparation of this manuscript. This research received no external funding.

Acknowledgments: We wish to thank Mireille Gerrits, of Terminal 4 Communications, Hilversum, the Netherlands for medical writing support.

Conflicts of Interest: D.F.A. owns stock or options in Agile Therapeutics and InnovaGyn, Inc., and is a consultant for AbbVie, Agile Therapeutics, Exeltis, Mayne Pharma, Mithra Pharmaceuticals, and TherapeuticsMD. Eastern Virginia Medical School receives research funding from AbbVie, Bayer Healthcare, Estetra SRL (an affiliate company of Mithra Pharmaceuticals), Myovant, ObsEva, and TherapeuticsMD. D.M. has received financial support to attend pharmaceutical advisory boards, speak at educational meetings/webinars/conferences, and undertake scientific research from Astellas, Bayer, Consilient Health, Gedeon Richter, HRA Pharma, MSD, Mithra, Organon, Pfizer, Viatris and Vifor Pharma. J.M.F. is co-founder of Mithra Pharmaceuticals, shareholder, and member of the Board.

References

1. Schrager, S. Abnormal uterine bleeding associated with hormonal contraception. *Am. Fam. Physician* **2002**, *65*, 2073–2080.
2. Villavicencio, J.; Allen, R.H. Unscheduled bleeding and contraceptive choice: Increasing satisfaction and continuation rates. *Open Access J. Contracept.* **2016**, *7*, 43–52. [CrossRef]
3. Rosenberg, M.J.; Waugh, M.S. Oral contraceptive discontinuation: A prospective evaluation of frequency and reasons. *Am. J. Obstet. Gynecol.* **1998**, *179*, 577–582. [CrossRef]
4. Rosenberg, M.J.; Long, S.C. Oral contraceptives and cycle control: A critical review of the literature. *Adv. Contracept.* **1992**, *8* (Suppl. S1), 35–45. [CrossRef]
5. Rosenberg, M.J.; Waugh, M.S.; Stevens, C.M. Smoking and cycle control among oral contraceptive users. *Am. J. Obstet. Gynecol.* **1996**, *174*, 628–632. [CrossRef]
6. Seif, M.W.; Diamond, K.; Nickkho-Amiry, M. Obesity and menstrual disorders. *Best Pract. Res. Clin. Obstet. Gynaecol.* **2015**, *29*, 516–527. [CrossRef]
7. Dinger, J.; Do Minh, T.; Heinemann, K. Impact of estrogen type on cardiovascular safety of combined oral contraceptives. *Contraception* **2016**, *94*, 328–339. [CrossRef]
8. Reed, S.; Koro, C.; DiBello, J.; Becker, K.; Bauerfeind, A.; Franke, C.; Heinemann, K. Prospective controlled cohort study on the safety of a monophasic oral contraceptive containing nomegestrol acetate (2.5 mg) and 17beta-oestradiol (1.5 mg) (PRO-E2 study): Risk of venous and arterial thromboembolism. *Eur. J. Contracept. Reprod. Health Care* **2021**, *26*, 439–446. [CrossRef]
9. Douxfils, J.; Klipping, C.; Duijkers, I.; Kinet, V.; Mawet, M.; Maillard, C.; Jost, M.; Rosing, J.; Foidart, J.M. Evaluation of the effect of a new oral contraceptive containing estetrol and drospirenone on hemostasis parameters. *Contraception* **2020**, *102*, 396–402. [CrossRef]
10. Bachmann, G.; Korner, P. Bleeding patterns associated with oral contraceptive use: A review of the literature. *Contraception* **2007**, *76*, 182–189. [CrossRef]
11. Belsey, E.M.; Machin, D.; d'Arcangues, C. The analysis of vaginal bleeding patterns induced by fertility regulating methods. World Health Organization Special Programme of Research, Development and Research Training in Human Reproduction. *Contraception* **1986**, *34*, 253–260. [CrossRef]

12. Mishell, D.R., Jr.; Guillebaud, J.; Westhoff, C.; Nelson, A.L.; Kaunitz, A.M.; Trussell, J.; Davis, A.J. Combined hormonal contraceptive trials: Variable data collection and bleeding assessment methodologies influence study outcomes and physician perception. *Contraception* **2007**, *75*, 4–10. [CrossRef] [PubMed]
13. Mishell, D.R., Jr.; Guillebaud, J.; Westhoff, C.; Nelson, A.L.; Kaunitz, A.M.; Trussell, J.; Davis, A.J. Recommendations for standardization of data collection and analysis of bleeding in combined hormone contraceptive trials. *Contraception* **2007**, *75*, 11–15. [CrossRef] [PubMed]
14. Hodkinson, A.; Dietz, K.C.; Lefebvre, C.; Golder, S.; Jones, M.; Doshi, P.; Heneghan, C.; Jefferson, T.; Boutron, I.; Stewart, L. The use of clinical study reports to enhance the quality of systematic reviews: A survey of systematic review authors. *Syst. Rev.* **2018**, *7*, 117. [CrossRef] [PubMed]
15. Clinicaltrials.gov. Available online: https://www.clinicaltrials.gov (accessed on 21 January 2022).
16. Nelson, A.; Parke, S.; Mellinger, U.; Zampaglione, E.; Schmidt, A. Efficacy and safety of a combined oral contraceptive containing estradiol valerate/dienogest: Results from a clinical study conducted in North America. *J. Womens Health* **2014**, *23*, 204–210. [CrossRef]
17. Center for Drug Evaluation and Research; Food and Drug Administration. Clinical Review Estradiol Valerate/Dienogest (NDA 22-252). 28 April 2010. Available online: https://www.accessdata.fda.gov/drugsatfda_docs/nda/2010/022252_Orig-1_MedR.pdf (accessed on 25 May 2022).
18. Palacios, S.; Wildt, L.; Parke, S.; Machlitt, A.; Romer, T.; Bitzer, J. Efficacy and safety of a novel oral contraceptive based on oestradiol (oestradiol valerate/dienogest): A Phase III trial. *Eur. J. Obstet. Gynecol. Reprod. Biol.* **2010**, *149*, 57–62. [CrossRef]
19. Apter, D.; Zimmerman, Y.; Beekman, L.; Mawet, M.; Maillard, C.; Foidart, J.M.; Bennink, H.J. Bleeding pattern and cycle control with estetrol-containing combined oral contraceptives: Results from a phase II, randomised, dose-finding study (FIESTA). *Contraception* **2016**, *94*, 366–373. [CrossRef]
20. Archer, D.F.; Nakajima, S.T.; Sawyer, A.T.; Wentworth, J.; Trupin, S.; Koltun, W.D.; Gilbert, R.D.; Ellman, H. Norethindrone acetate 1.0 milligram and ethinyl estradiol 10 micrograms as an ultra low-dose oral contraceptive. *Obstet. Gynecol.* **2013**, *122*, 601–607. [CrossRef]
21. FDA. Medical Review Lo Loestrin (NDA 22-501). 4 October 2010. Available online: https://www.accessdata.fda.gov/drugsatfda_docs/nda/2010/022501Orig1s000MedR.pdf (accessed on 25 May 2022).
22. Mansour, D.; Verhoeven, C.; Sommer, W.; Weisberg, E.; Taneepanichskul, S.; Melis, G.B.; Sundstrom-Poromaa, I.; Korver, T. Efficacy and tolerability of a monophasic combined oral contraceptive containing nomegestrol acetate and 17beta-oestradiol in a 24/4 regimen, in comparison to an oral contraceptive containing ethinylestradiol and drospirenone in a 21/7 regimen. *Eur. J. Contracept. Reprod. Health Care* **2011**, *16*, 430–443. [CrossRef]
23. Australian Government, Department of Health and Ageing Therapeutic Goods Administration. Australian Public Assessment Report for Nomegestrol Acetate/Oestradiol. October 2011. Available online: https://www.tga.gov.au/sites/default/files/auspar-zoely.pdf (accessed on 25 May 2022).
24. Westhoff, C.; Kaunitz, A.M.; Korver, T.; Sommer, W.; Bahamondes, L.; Darney, P.; Verhoeven, C. Efficacy, safety, and tolerability of a monophasic oral contraceptive containing nomegestrol acetate and 17beta-estradiol: A randomized controlled trial. *Obstet. Gynecol.* **2012**, *119*, 989–999. [CrossRef]
25. Mansour, D.; Westhoff, C.; Kher, U.; Korver, T. Pooled analysis of two randomized, open-label studies comparing the effects of nomegestrol acetate/17beta-estradiol and drospirenone/ethinyl estradiol on bleeding patterns in healthy women. *Contraception* **2017**, *95*, 390–397. [CrossRef] [PubMed]
26. Gemzell-Danielsson, K.; Apter, D.; Zatik, J.; Weyers, S.; Piltonen, T.; Suturina, L.; Apolikhina, I.; Jost, M.; Creinin, M.D.; Foidart, J.M. Estetrol-Drospirenone combination oral contraceptive: A clinical study of contraceptive efficacy, bleeding pattern and safety in Europe and Russia. *BJOG* **2022**, *129*, 63–71. [CrossRef] [PubMed]
27. Center for Drug Evaluation and Research; Food and Drug Administration. Multi-Discipline Review of Nextstellis (NDA 214154). 15 April 2021. Available online: https://www.fda.gov/media/149979/download (accessed on 25 May 2022).
28. Creinin, M.D.; Westhoff, C.L.; Bouchard, C.; Chen, M.J.; Jensen, J.T.; Kaunitz, A.M.; Achilles, S.L.; Foidart, J.M.; Archer, D.F. Estetrol-drospirenone combination oral contraceptive: North American phase 3 efficacy and safety results. *Contraception* **2021**, *104*, 222–228. [CrossRef] [PubMed]
29. Archer, D.F.; Ahrendt, H.J.; Drouin, D. Drospirenone-only oral contraceptive: Results from a multicenter noncomparative trial of efficacy, safety and tolerability. *Contraception* **2015**, *92*, 439–444. [CrossRef] [PubMed]
30. Center for Drug Evaluation and Research; Food and Drug Administration. Multi-Disciplinary Review and Evaluation Slynd (NDA 211367). 24 May 2019. Available online: https://www.fda.gov/media/129539/download (accessed on 25 May 2022).
31. Palacios, S.; Colli, E.; Regidor, P.A. Bleeding profile of women using a drospirenone-only pill 4 mg over nine cycles in comparison with desogestrel 0.075 mg. *PLoS ONE* **2020**, *15*, e0231856. [CrossRef]
32. Kimble, T.; Burke, A.E.; Barnhart, K.T.; Archer, D.F.; Colli, E.; Westhoff, C.L. A 1-year prospective, open-label, single-arm, multicenter, phase 3 trial of the contraceptive efficacy and safety of the oral progestin-only pill drospirenone 4 mg using a 24/4-day regimen. *Contracept. X* **2020**, *2*, 100020. [CrossRef]
33. Australian Government, Department of Health and Ageing Therapeutic Goods Administration. Australian Public Assessment Report for Nomegestrol Acetate/Oestradiol (Zoely). October 2011. Available online: https://www.tga.gov.au/sites/default/files/auspar-zoely.pdf (accessed on 25 May 2022).

34. Center for Drug Evaluation and Research; Food and Drug Administration. Medical Review Yaz (NDA 21-676). 16 May 2006. Available online: https://www.accessdata.fda.gov/drugsatfda_docs/nda/2006/021676s000_MEDR_pt1.pdf (accessed on 25 May 2022).
35. Bachmann, G.; Sulak, P.J.; Sampson-Landers, C.; Benda, N.; Marr, J. Efficacy and safety of a low-dose 24-day combined oral contraceptive containing 20 micrograms ethinylestradiol and 3 mg drospirenone. *Contraception* **2004**, *70*, 191–198. [CrossRef]
36. Ahrendt, H.J.; Makalova, D.; Parke, S.; Mellinger, U.; Mansour, D. Bleeding pattern and cycle control with an estradiol-based oral contraceptive: A seven-cycle, randomized comparative trial of estradiol valerate/dienogest and ethinyl estradiol/levonorgestrel. *Contraception* **2009**, *80*, 436–444. [CrossRef]
37. Hagen, A.A.; Barr, M.; Diczfalusy, E. Metabolism of 17-Beta-Oestradiol-4-14-C in Early Infancy. *Acta Endocrinol.* **1965**, *49*, 207–220. [CrossRef]
38. Warmerdam, E.G.; Visser, M.; Coelingh Bennink, H.J.; Groen, M. A new route of synthesis of estetrol. *Climacteric* **2008**, *11* (Suppl. S1), 59–63. [CrossRef]
39. Gérard, C.; Arnal, J.F.; Jost, M.; Douxfils, J.; Lenfant, F.; Fontaine, C.; Houtman, R.; Archer, D.F.; Reid, R.L.; Lobo, R.A.; et al. Profile of estetrol, a promising native estrogen for oral contraception and the relief of climacteric symptoms of menopause. *Expert. Rev. Clin. Pharmacol.* **2022**, *15*, 121–137. [CrossRef] [PubMed]
40. Fruzzetti, F.; Fidecicchi, T.; Montt Guevara, M.M.; Simoncini, T. Estetrol: A New Choice for Contraception. *J. Clin. Med.* **2021**, *10*, 5625. [CrossRef]
41. Creinin, M.D.; Vieira, C.S.; Westhoff, C.L.; Mansour, D.J.A. Recommendations for standardization of bleeding data analyses in contraceptive studies. *Contraception* **2022**, *112*, 14–22. [CrossRef] [PubMed]
42. Gallo, M.F.; Nanda, K.; Grimes, D.A.; Lopez, L.M.; Schulz, K.F. 20 microg versus >20 microg estrogen combined oral contraceptives for contraception. *Cochrane Database Syst. Rev.* **2013**, *8*, CD003989. [CrossRef]
43. Blode, H.; Kowal, K.; Roth, K.; Reif, S. Pharmacokinetics of drospirenone and ethinylestradiol in Caucasian and Japanese women. *Eur. J. Contracept. Reprod. Health Care* **2012**, *17*, 284–297. [CrossRef]
44. Gerrits, M.G.; Schnabel, P.G.; Post, T.M.; Peeters, P.A. Pharmacokinetic profile of nomegestrol acetate and 17beta-estradiol after multiple and single dosing in healthy women. *Contraception* **2013**, *87*, 193–200. [CrossRef]
45. Polis, C.B.; Hussain, R.; Berry, A. There might be blood: A scoping review on women's responses to contraceptive-induced menstrual bleeding changes. *Reprod. Health* **2018**, *15*, 114. [CrossRef]
46. Wiegratz, I.; Hommel, H.H.; Zimmermann, T.; Kuhl, H. Attitude of German women and gynecologists towards long-cycle treatment with oral contraceptives. *Contraception* **2004**, *69*, 37–42. [CrossRef]

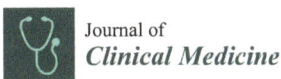

Article

Norethisterone Reduces Vaginal Bleeding Caused by Progesterone-Only Birth Control Pills

Naama Vilk Ayalon [1,†], Lior Segev [2,3,*,†], Abraham O. Samson [4], Simcha Yagel [1], Sarah M. Cohen [1], Tamar Green [5] and Hila Hochler [1,*]

1 Department of Obstetrics and Gynecology, Hadassah Medical Center, Faculty of Medicine, Hebrew University of Jerusalem, Jerusalem 9190401, Israel; naamaayalon@gmail.com (N.V.A.); simcha.yagel@gmail.com (S.Y.); sarahc362@gmail.com (S.M.C.)
2 Science and Halacha Program, General History Department, Bar-Ilan University, Ramat-Gan 5290002, Israel
3 Puah Institute, Jerusalem 9547735, Israel
4 Faculty of Medicine, Bar-Ilan University, Safed 1311502, Israel; avraham.samson@biu.ac.il
5 Department of Obstetrics and Gynecology, Shaare Zedek Medical Center, Jerusalem 9103102, Israel; tamargreen1@gmail.com
* Correspondence: segevyl@gmail.com (L.S.); hilahochler@gmail.com (H.H.); Tel.: +972-2-5844511 (H.H.)
† These authors contributed equally to this work.

Abstract: (1) Background: Progesterone-only pills (POP) are widely used contraceptives. About 40% of women taking these pills report vaginal bleeding/spotting; 25% find this a reason for cessation. To date, no effective remedy has been described. We aimed to examine the therapeutic approaches offered by health providers. (2) Methods: A prospective questionnaire-based study of women experiencing vaginal bleeding due to POP, comparing the effectiveness of prescribed therapies. Women were recruited through social networks, and subsequently divided into groups according to the treatment offered: (1) POP with norethisterone ($n = 36$); (2) double dose POP ($n = 19$); (3) single dose POP (continuing initial treatment, $n = 57$); and (4) different POP formula ($n = 8$). Women rated bleeding quantity and frequency at four intervals, at weeks 0, 2, 4, and 6. (3) Results: Women who added 5 mg norethisterone acetate reported a significant decrease in bleeding frequency compared to the other groups, observed after 2, 4, and 6 weeks (p-values 0.019, 0.002, and 0.002, respectively). Women also reported an overall decrease in combined bleeding quantity and frequency (p-values 0.028, 0.003, and 0.005, respectively). There was no difference in the rate of side effects among groups. (4) Conclusions: Adding 5 mg norethisterone acetate (Primolut-nor) to progesterone-only pills significantly reduces bleeding and spotting associated with POP contraception.

Keywords: norethisterone acetate; POP; progesterone-only pills; vaginal bleeding; vaginal spotting; contraception

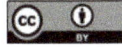

1. Introduction

Progesterone-only pills (POP) are widely used contraceptive agents, in particular by lactating women [1]. A substantial proportion of POP users—up to 40%—report spotting or irregular bleeding while on the pill [2]. Moreover, irregular bleeding and spotting are the main reason for discontinued POP use, and reportedly 25% of users stop using hormonal contraceptives due to irregular bleeding [3].

To resolve unscheduled bleeding associated with POP, several treatments have been proposed. Danielsson et al., reported a decrease in bleeding patterns when using antiprogestogen with POPs [4], although reanalysis of their data did not reveal any efficacy [5]. A very small study administering ethinylestradiol found no benefit [6]. Doubling the dose or switching the type of POPs have also been proposed; however, these approaches were also not shown to be effective [7]. Therefore, the Royal College of Obstetrics and Gynecology (RCOG) concludes that to date there are no effective treatments for this problem [8]. In clinical practice, some caregivers prescribe norethisterone acetate to reduce bleeding. To the best of our knowledge, this practice had not yet been tested.

In this study, we examine the effect of therapeutic approaches offered by health providers to treat menstrual irregularity associated with POP via an online questionnaire.

2. Materials and Methods

Women were recruited through social networks—Facebook groups aimed toward pregnant and lactating women, as well as the client mailing list of the Puah Institute, Jerusalem, Israel, which is a medical-halachic institute in Israel. Eligible participants were breastfeeding women up to six months after delivery, who experience irregular bleeding associated to POP. Exclusion criteria were switching to combined contraceptive pills, or failing to complete all questionnaires.

Recruited patients had been examined by their attending physician regarding medical history, to exclude other potential causes of their complaint and determine management.

Patients completed four online questionnaires. The first questionnaire (Appendix A) included questions about the socioeconomic status, medical background, the type of POP used, and questions characterizing the quantity and frequency of bleeding associated with the treatment offered to reduce irregular bleeding. This study did not include parity, and only measured the time from last delivery.

Women who met inclusion criteria were asked to complete three more follow-up questionnaires, two, four, and six weeks after the first one. In order to monitor bleeding patterns over time, and to improve the participant response rate, we used a biweekly questionnaire rather than the previously used daily one [9]. As such, we prepared a biweekly questionnaire based on existing recommendations for assessing bleeding under hormonal contraceptives [9]. These three follow-up questionnaires were identical (Appendix A) and asked women to rate the quantity and frequency of bleeding, as well as side effects of the treatment. The quantity of bleeding was measured using a five-point Likert scale, while the frequency was measured on a seven-point Likert scale, as detailed in Appendix A. Before statistical analysis, we translated both measurements to a scale of 10 [10].

This study was approved by the Ethics Committee of the Institutional Review Board (IRB permit 3.11.19) of Bar-Ilan University and was conducted between March 2019 and March 2020 in Israel.

Participants reported four treatments prescribed by their gynecologists to treat menstrual irregularity; they were categorized to four groups based on these responses:

(1) single dose POP (control, $n = 57$), (2) double dose POP ($n = 19$), (3) different POP formulation ($n = 8$), and (4) POP with norethisterone ($n = 36$). Women who received norethisterone were asked to stop treatment for 5 days, prior to adding norethisterone (Primolut-nor, 5 mg) in combination with POP.

Statistical Analysis

To examine the effects of different treatments on bleeding patterns, we calculated the difference in the quantity and frequency of bleeding between the initial questionnaire and the three follow-up questionnaires, for each participant individually. In addition, we defined a variable combining frequency and quantity (with each variable weighted equally). Data analysis was carried out after translating the five- and seven-point Likert scale responses to a ten-point scale, according to orderly transformations [10].

We compared categorical variables using Chi-square or Fisher exact tests, according to the distribution of expected frequencies. According to the variable distribution and sample size, relationships between quantitative/ordinal variables were analyzed by Pearson or Spearman tests.

Differences between study groups were examined by t-test or by analysis of variance (ANOVA). If the ANOVA tests were statistically significant, we performed a multiple comparison applying the Benjamini–Hochberg procedure to control the false discovery rate (FDR) at a level of alpha = 0.05. Differences in ordinal variables were analyzed by Mann–

Whitney or Kruskal–Wallis tests. Friedman test was performed to analyze the differences in bleeding rates between different questionnaires.

Statistical analysis was performed using the SPSS program, version 25.0. Statistical significance was determined as $p < 0.05$, and all tests were two-tailed. If the results of the parametric or asymmetric variance analysis tests were statistically significant, Bonferroni's correction for multiple analyses was applied to control Type-I error.

3. Results
3.1. Demographics and Baseline Characteristics

The first questionnaire was answered by 174 patients. Excluded cases comprised 43 who did not complete all the questionnaires (37 failed to complete one questionnaire, 6 failed to complete two or more), five who reported no bleeding or spotting, and six who were using other forms of contraception concomitantly with POP.

Thus, a total of 120 women were included in the study. The vast majority of women (77%) reported use of Desogestrel 0.075 mg (Diamilla, Fominic, and Cerazette), while 23% reported use of Levonorgestrel 30 mcg (Microlut).

Women reported four different prescription treatments to treat menstrual irregularity and bleeding: (1) adding 5 mg norethisterone acetate (Primolut-Nor) after a five-day pause in taking the POP ($n = 36$), (2) doubling the POP dose ($n = 19$), (3) continuing using POP as before ($n = 57$), and (4) changing to another formulation of POP ($n = 8$).

The demographic and baseline characteristics of women taking each of these treatments were similar statistically, and their ages ranged from 20 to 44 years (Table 1). Notably, only eight women changed the POPs to another brand, which was a relatively small group compared to the other treatment groups, and disrupted the statistical comparison. As a result, this small group of women was omitted from our data analysis.

Table 1. Baseline demographic and obstetric characteristics of the study participants.

	Group 1 Norethisterone Acetate	Group 2 Doubling Dose	Group 3 No Change	Group 4 Switching Type	*p*-Value
N	36	19	57	8	
POP TYPE					
Desogestrel	29	14	42	8	0.18
Levonorgestrel	7	5	15	0	
AGE					
Mean ± SD	28 ± 5	26 ± 5	27 ± 5	28 ± 5	0.45
EDUCATION					
Non-academic	3	1	5	3	0.21
Academic	32	13	52	5	
DELIVERY					
Vaginal delivery	34	16	52	5	0.12
Cesarean section	2	3	5	3	
BREASTFEEDING					
Full	31	15	52	7	0.58
Partial	5	4	5	1	

3.2. Treatment Response

Women who added 5 mg of norethisterone acetate to POP contraception reported a significant reduction in the frequency of bleeding compared to the other treatment groups after 2, 4, and 6 weeks of treatment (Table 2). In addition, these women reported more days of bleeding prior to treatment, emphasizing the results. This reduction in bleeding frequency was particularly pronounced in the comparison between women that added norethisterone acetate (group 1) and those who used a single dose POP (group 3, control).

Table 2. Comparison of bleeding frequency (mean ± SD).

		Group 1 Adding Norethisterone Acetate	Group 2 Doubling Dose	Group 3 No Change	p-Value *
Bleeding frequency at baseline (first questionnaire) on a scale of 10 [X]		3.7 (±0.8)	3.2 (±1.3)	2.6 (±1.5)	0.001 [1]
Difference from baseline to:	2 weeks	7.0 (±4.3)	4.6 (±4.5)	5.2 (±4.1)	0.019 [2]
	4 weeks	8 (±3.78)	4.4 (±4.6)	4.8 (±4.8)	0.004 [3]
	6 weeks	7.9 (±3.17)	5.4 (±4.5)	4.8 (±4.2)	0.002 [4]

[X] Data analysis was conducted by correcting the five-and seven-point Likert scale responses to a ten-point scale of infrequency. * p value by Kruskal–Wallis (First questionnaire) and by one-way ANOVA (Subsequent questionnaires). [1] A significant difference between groups 1 and 3 (p = 0.001). [2] A significant difference between groups 1 and 3 (p = 0.019). [3] A significant difference between groups 1 and 3 (p = 0.004), and also between groups 1 and 2 (p = 0.0021). [4] A significant difference between groups 1 and 3 (p = 0.002).

In addition, adding norethisterone acetate resulted in a greater reduction in bleeding quantity, measured as the change in bleeding quantity between the first and the three subsequent questionnaires. Inconclusively, however, the comparison between different treatments was not statistically significant (Table 3).

Table 3. Comparison of bleeding quantity (mean ± SD).

		Group 1 Adding Norethisterone Acetate	Group 2 Doubling the Dose	Group 3 No Change	p-Value *
Bleeding Quantity at baseline (questionnaire 1) on a scale of 10 [X]		4.3 ± 1.7	1.6 ± 4.1	4.0 ± 1.6	0.703 [1]
Difference from baseline to:	2 weeks	5.97 ± 3.39	3.75 ± 4.65	5.03 ± 3.25	0.294 [2]
	4 weeks	6.57 ± 3.33	4.35 ± 4.99	5.19 ± 3.56	0.091 [3]
	6 weeks	6.72 ± 2.86	5.39 ± 4.66	5.52 ± 3.29	0.246 [4]

[X] Data analysis was conducted by correcting the five-and seven-point Likert scale responses to a ten-point scale of inverse quantity. * p value by Kruskal–Wallis (First questionnaire) and by one-way ANOVA (Subsequent questionnaires). [1] Insignificant difference between groups 1 and 3 (p = 0.703). [2] Insignificant difference between groups 1 and 3 (p = 0.294). [3] Insignificant difference between groups 1 and 3 (p = 0.094). [4] Insignificant difference between groups 1 and 3 (p = 0.246).

A variable combining frequency and quantity of bleeding (with each variable weighted equally) also decreased when norethisterone acetate was prescribed, as compared to the other groups (Table 4). Notably, the reduction was statistically significant at each subsequent follow-up.

Table 5 shows side effects as reported by women in the fourth questionnaire, 6 weeks after starting the treatment. We found no significant difference in side effects throughout the study. Furthermore, participants were asked directly about the impact of the treatment on breastfeeding, and here also no significant difference was reported.

Table 4. Comparison of combined frequency and quantity.

		Group 1 Adding Norethisterone Acetate	Group 2 Doubling the Dose	Group 3 No Change	p-Value *
Combined frequency and quantity at baseline (questionnaire 1) on a scale of 10 ^{X}		8.17 ± 2.07	7.37 ± 2.11	6.60 ± 2.34	0.122 [1]
Difference from baseline to:	2 weeks	6.49 ± 3.49	4.63 ± 3.61	4.52 ± 3.51	0.028 [2]
	4 weeks	7.29 ± 3.25	4.40 ± 4.28	4.90 ± 3.39	0.003 [3]
	6 weeks	7.33 ± 2.59	5.42 ± 3.97	5.09 ± 2.88	0.005 [4]

^{X} Data analysis was conducted by correcting the five-and seven-point Likert scale responses to a ten-point scale of inverse quantity. * p value by Kruskal–Wallis (First questionnaire) and by one-way ANOVA (Subsequent questionnaires). [1] Significant difference between groups 1 and 3 (p = 0.028). [2] Significant difference between groups 1 and 3 (p = 0.003). [3] Significant difference between groups 1 and 3 (p = 0.005). [4] Insignificant difference between groups 1 and 3 (p = 0.246).

Table 5. Side effects at six weeks.

	Group 1 Norethisterone Acetate 5 mg	Group 2 Doubling Dose	Group 3 No Change	Group 4 Switching Type	p-Value
No adverse effect	26 (77%)	14 (82%)	39 (85%)	5 (83%)	
Decreased libido	4 (12%)	0 (0%)	2 (4%)	0 (0%)	0.198
Headache/abdominal pain/dizziness	0 (0%)	0 (0%)	1 (2%)	0 (0%)	
Mood swings/depression/fatigue	3 (9%)	2 (12%)	2 (4%)	1 (17%)	
No change in breastfeeding	25 (73%)	12 (70%)	43 (94%)	5 (83%)	
Decreased in breastfeeding	8 (24%)	3 (18%)	3 (6%)	1 (17%)	0.083
Stopped breastfeeding	1 (3%)	2 (11%)	0 (0%)	0 (0%)	

4. Discussion

Our study focused on resolving vaginal bleeding and spotting through the use of POP. Adding norethisterone acetate to POP after a five-day pause in taking the POP led to a reduction in bleeding, as compared to single and double POP doses. Women who used norethisterone acetate did not report any additional side effects.

We are aware of only three previous studies which examined treatments for vaginal bleeding caused by POP use. The largest and most recent of these [4] included 103 women and examined the addition of antiprogesterone (Org 31,710) vs. placebo once every 28 days. The authors found improvement in the bleeding profile; nonetheless, women continued to bleed every month, and the effectiveness of the treatment decreased over time. Notably, Org 31,710 is currently not marketed, and a reanalysis of the data showed no benefit [5]. The treatment, though effective, was based on a small cohort (20 women in the intervention group, both POP and IUD users), and required prolonged treatment (20 continuous days every month). Another study [6] examined 50 µg ethinylestradiol for 7 days vs. placebo. The cohort included only 12 women and the investigators found no benefit using this treatment. Indeed, the RCOG [7] indicates a lack of evidence for an effective treatment of bleeding in women using POP.

Few other studies have examined the effectiveness of different treatments on long term POP contraceptives, including injection of depot medroxyprogesterone acetate, subdermal etonogestrel, as well as levonorgestrel implants and intrauterine devices [5,11]. Treatments used were mifepristone, tranexamic acid, and NSAIDs, with conflicting results. We did not find studies that examined these treatments on POP users. In addition, these studies do not necessarily apply to POP, since other contraceptives were based on different progestin types and have different mechanisms of action.

As a potential limitation to this study, the mechanism of action of norethisterone acetate is not well understood. We hypothesize that its effect is based on its partial metabolism to ethinylestradiol in vivo. This metabolism was first reported in 1960 by Breuer and colleagues [12], who detected ethinylestradiol in the urine of women receiving norethisterone. Supporting evidence was provided by later in vitro studies in human placental microsomes, in homogenate of human liver, and in human hepatocytes [13–15]. Another study has examined the metabolism of norethisterone acetate and found that its metabolites bind to the human estrogen receptors [16].

Additionally, while the majority of women in this study received desogestrel, about one-quarter received levonorgestrel. We did not control for this variation in progesterone formulation.

Further studies in humans have attempted to estimate the conversion ratio of norethisterone acetate to ethinylestradiol. One study in 24 postmenopausal women who received norethisterone acetate 5 or 10 mg every morning found that every 5 mg of oral norethisterone acetate (one pill of Primolut-Nor) is equivalent to 28.1 ± 7.1 µg ethinylestradiol, and 10 mg norethisterone acetate is equivalent to 62.4 ± 18.6 µg ethinylestradiol [17]. In another study of 20 premenopausal women who received 10, 20, or 40 mg of norethisterone acetate daily for 7 days in the early follicular phase, the authors estimated the conversion ratio to be between 0.2% and 0.33%, which means that every 5 mg of oral norethisterone acetate is equivalent to 7.5 µg ethinylestradiol [18].

We hypothesize that the metabolite ethinylestradiol may have a beneficial effect on vaginal bleeding. It is well-known that exogenous estrogen may aid in tissue repair and stabilization of the endometrial lining [11]. It is thus plausible that norethindrone acetate works similarly in reducing bleeding. As mentioned above, the study that examined ethinylestradiol to treat vaginal bleeding due to POP showed no significant benefit [6]. Nevertheless, this might be due to the different dosage and the very small cohort of 12 women.

It is important to note that use of norethisterone acetate, which metabolizes into ethinylestradiol, warrants caution, especially in women with increased risk for thromboembolism or with other contraindications to exogenous estrogen [19].

Additionally, the conversion into ethinyl estradiol raises the question of prescribing combined oral contraception to breastfeeding women, which is a controversial issue [20,21]. We note that there are inconsistent data about the hormonal effects on milk quality and quantity, and about the passage of hormones to the infant. As a result, major organizations have adopted different recommendations: the WHO [22] and the RCOG [23] advise delaying use of combined oral contraceptives until 6 months postpartum for women who are primarily breastfeeding. In contrast, the CDC [24] allows the initiation of estrogen-containing contraceptive methods 6 weeks postpartum. Adding norethindrone to POP reportedly does not adversely affect the composition or the production of milk [25], and the passage of norethisterone acetate into nursing infants is expected to be minimal. It is likely that norethisterone acetate is also safe during lactation, although the manufacturer recommends cautionary use. In our study, we did not find more side effects on breastfeeding with norethisterone acetate compared to the other groups.

To the best of our knowledge, this is the first study to describe an effective treatment for unscheduled intermittent vaginal bleeding with POP. This is also the first report of norethisterone acetate to treat irregular bleeding during POP use. Our findings provide a useful strategy to reduce the bleeding profile of POP users. Since one of the main reasons for discontinuing POP is irregular bleeding and spotting, our findings may improve compliance and continuation rates, as well as patient satisfaction with POP.

Despite these encouraging results, this study has several limitations. First, this study is observational, and thus there might be a bias in the assigned groups and in the initial characteristics of women who added norethindrone acetate. Second, we used nonvalidated questionnaires.

To further confirm our results, additional studies may be required; for example, a prospective study to assess the effectiveness of norethindrone acetate compared to placebo and other treatments mentioned (e.g., mifepristone, tranexamic acid, and NSAIDs), as well as basic research to understand the exact mechanism of action of norethisterone acetate in reducing vaginal bleeding with POPs.

5. Conclusions

For women suffering from irregular vaginal bleeding associated with POP use, adding 5 mg norethisterone acetate (Primolut-Nor) after a five-day pause in taking the POP effectively reduces bleeding, without additional side effects.

Author Contributions: Conceptualization, L.S. and H.H.; Data curation, L.S.; Formal analysis, L.S. and H.H.; Investigation, L.S., T.G. and H.H.; Methodology, L.S. and H.H.; Project administration, L.S., T.G. and H.H.; Supervision, S.Y. and H.H.; Validation, L.S.; Writing—original draft, N.V.A., S.M.C. and H.H.; Writing – review & editing, L.S., A.O.S. and S.M.C. All authors have read and agreed to the published version of the manuscript.

Funding: This research received no external funding.

Institutional Review Board Statement: This study was approved by the Ethics Committee of the Institutional Review Board (IRB 3.11.19) of Bar-Ilan University and was conducted between March 2019 and March 2020 in Israel.

Informed Consent Statement: Informed consent was obtained from all subjects involved in the study.

Data Availability Statement: Not applicable.

Conflicts of Interest: The authors declare no conflict of interest.

Appendix A

The questionnaires

The first questionnaire

- Age
- Occupation
- Education

  Elementary school
  High school
  Academic

- Date of last delivery
- Vaginal delivery or cesarean section
- How many weeks after delivery did your vaginal bleeding stop?
- Partial breastfeeding or full breastfeeding
- Type of pill:

  Diamilla, Fominic, Cerazette, Microlut, other

- Amount of bleeding (Two weeks after the first pill)

  0. No vaginal bleeding
  1. Very light spotting
  2. Spotting up to 2 cm a day
  3. Spotting up to a quarter of a pantyliners a day
  4. Spotting between a quarter of a pantyliner and a pad a day.
  5. Less than a period
  6. A period or more

- How many days after first pill did the bleeding start?

- Frequency of bleeding (Two weeks after the first pill)
    0. No vaginal bleeding
    1. Less than once a week
    2. Up to four times a week
    3. Once a day
    4. Multiple times a day
- What treatment did your doctor offer?

The follow-up questionnaire (questionnaires 2–4)
- Amount of bleeding 2/4/6 weeks after starting treatment:
    0. No vaginal bleeding
    1. Very light spotting
    2. Spotting up to 2 cm a day
    3. Spotting up to a quarter of a pantyliners a day
    4. Spotting between a quarter of a pantyliner and a pad a day.
    5. Less than a period
    6. A period or more
- Frequency of bleeding 2/4/6 weeks after starting treatment:
    0. No vaginal bleeding
    1. Less than once a week
    2. Up to four times a week
    3. Once a day
    4. Multiple times a day
- Did you have side effects because of the treatment? If so, please describe them.
- Did the treatment affect breastfeeding? If so, please elaborate.

References

1. Howie, P.W. The Progestogen-Only Pill. *Br. J. Obstet. Gynaecol.* **1985**, *92*, 1001–1002. [CrossRef] [PubMed]
2. Belsey, E. Vaginal Bleeding Patterns among Women Using One Natural and Eight Hormonal Methods of Contraception. *Contraception* **1988**, *38*, 181–206. [CrossRef]
3. Diedrich, J.T.; Zhao, Q.; Madden, T.; Secura, G.M.; Peipert, J.F. Three-Year Continuation of Reversible Contraception. *Am. J. Obstet. Gynecol.* **2015**, *213*, 662.e1–662.e8. [CrossRef] [PubMed]
4. Gemzell-Danielsson, K.; van Heusden, A.M.; Killick, S.R.; Croxatto, H.B.; Bouchard, P.; Cameron, S.; Bygdeman, M. Improving Cycle Control in Progestogen-Only Contraceptive Pill Users by Intermittent Treatment with a New Anti-Progestogen. *Hum. Reprod.* **2002**, *17*, 2588–2593. [CrossRef] [PubMed]
5. Abdel-Aleem, H.; d'Arcangues, C.; Vogelsong, K.M.; Gaffield, M.L.; Gülmezoglu, A.M. Treatment of Vaginal Bleeding Irregularities Induced by Progestin Only Contraceptives. *Cochrane Database Syst. Rev.* **2013**, *2013*, CD003449. [CrossRef]
6. Monteil-Seurin, J.; Bernard-Fernier, M.F.; Martinaggi, P.; Demarez, J.P.; Cauquil, J.; Lafont, A. Evaluation of the Efficacy of a Venotonic Capillary Protector in the Treatment of Metrorrhagia Due to IUD or Micropill Contraception. *Contracept. Fertil. Sex.* **1985**, *13*, 721–725.
7. Johannisson, E.; Landgren, B.-M.; Diczfalusy, E. Endometrial Morphology And Peripheral Steroid Levels In Women With And Without Intermenstrual Bleeding During Contraception With The 300 Ug Norethisterone (Net) Minipill. *Contraception* **1982**, *25*, 13–30. [CrossRef]
8. Faculty of Sexual and Reproductive Healthcare. *Faculty of Sexual & Reproductive Healthcare Clinical Guidance Management of Unscheduled Bleeding in Women Using Hormonal Contraception Clinical Effectiveness Unit*; RCOG: London, UK, 2009.
9. Mishell, D.R.; Guillebaud, J.; Westhoff, C.; Nelson, A.L.; Kaunitz, A.M.; Trussell, J.; Davis, A.J. Recommendations for Standardization of Data Collection and Analysis of Bleeding in Combined Hormone Contraceptive Trials. *Contraception* **2007**, *75*, 11–15. [CrossRef]
10. Marshall, A.W.; William, D.; Jean-Baptiste, R.; Wets, R. Order-preserving functions: Applications to majorization and order statistics. *Pac. J. Math.* **1967**, *23*, 569–584. [CrossRef]
11. Zigler, R.E.; McNicholas, C. Unscheduled Vaginal Bleeding with Progestin-Only Contraceptive Use. *Am. J. Obstet. Gynecol.* **2017**, *216*, 443–450. [CrossRef]
12. Breuer, H.; Dardenne, U.; Nocke, W. Excretion of 17-Ketosteroids, 17-Ketogenic Steroids and Estrogens in Man after the Administration of 17 Alpha-Ethynyl-19-Nortestosterone Esters. *Acta Endocrinol.* **1960**, *33*, 10–26. [CrossRef]
13. Barbieri, R.L.; Petro, Z.; Canick, J.A.; Ryan, K.J. Aromatization of Norethindrone to Ethinyl Estradiol by Human Placental Microsomes *. *J. Clin. Endocrinol. Metab.* **1983**, *57*, 299–303. [CrossRef] [PubMed]

14. Yamamoto, T.; Yoshiji, S.; Yasuda, J.; Shiroshita, K.; Kitawaki, J.; Fujii, M.; Urabe, M.; Honjo, H.; Okada, H. Aromatization of Norethindrone to Ethynylestradiol in Human Adult Liver. *Endocrinol. Jpn.* **1986**, *33*, 527–531. [CrossRef] [PubMed]
15. Yamamoto, T.; Kitawaki, J.; Shiroshita, K.; Urabe, M.; Sasaki, J.; Fukuoka, M.; Naitoh, K.; Honjo, H.; Okada, H. The Confirmation of Norethindrone Aromatization in Primary Human Hepatocytes by the Vitafiber-II Cell Culture System. *Nihon Sanka Fujinka Gakkai Zasshi* **1988**, *40*, 87–89. [PubMed]
16. Pasapera, A.M.; Gutiérrez-Sagal, R.; Herrera, J.; Galicia-Canales, N.; García de la Mora, G.; Ulloa-Aguirre, A. Norethisterone Is Bioconverted to Oestrogenic Compounds That Activate Both the Oestrogen Receptor α and Oestrogen Receptor β In Vitro. *Eur. J. Pharmacol.* **2002**, *452*, 347–355. [CrossRef]
17. Kuhnz, W.; Heuner, A.; Hiimpel, M.; Seifert, W.; Michaelist, K. In vivo Conversion of Norethisterone and Norethisterone Acetate to Ethinyl Etradiol in Postmenopausal Women. *Contraception* **1997**, *56*, 379–385. [CrossRef]
18. Chu, M.C.; Zhang, X.; Gentzschein, E.; Stanczyk, F.Z.; Lobo, R.A. Formation of Ethinyl Estradiol in Women during Treatment with Norethindrone Acetate. *J. Clin. Endocrinol. Metab.* **2007**, *92*, 2205–2207. [CrossRef]
19. Mansour, D. Safer Prescribing of Therapeutic Norethisterone for Women at Risk of Venous Thromboembolism. *J. Fam. Plan. Reprod. Health Care* **2012**, *38*, 148–149. [CrossRef]
20. Lopez, L.M.; Grey, T.W.; Stuebe, A.M.; Chen, M.; Truitt, S.T.; Gallo, M.F. Combined Hormonal versus Nonhormonal versus Progestin-Only Contraception in Lactation. *Cochrane Database Syst. Rev.* **2015**, *3*, CD003988. [CrossRef]
21. Bahamondes, L.; Bahamondes, M.V.; Modesto, W.; Tilley, I.B.; Magalhães, A.; Pinto e Silva, J.L.; Amaral, E.; Mishell, D.R. Effect of Hormonal Contraceptives during Breastfeeding on Infant's Milk Ingestion and Growth. *Fertil. Steril.* **2013**, *100*, 445–450. [CrossRef]
22. World Health Organization. *Medical Eligibility Criteria for Contraceptive Use*; WHO: Geneve, Swtizerland, 2015; ISBN 9789241549158.
23. Welsh, A. *Best Practice in Postpartum Family Planning*; RCOG: London, UK, 2015.
24. Curtis, K.M.; Tepper, N.K.; Jatlaoui, T.C.; Berry-Bibee, E.; Horton, L.G.; Zapata, L.B.; Simmons, K.B.; Pagano, H.P.; Jamieson, D.J.; Whiteman, M.K. U.S. Medical Eligibility Criteria for Contraceptive Use, 2016. *Morb. Mortal. Wkly. Rep. Recomm. Rep.* **2016**, *65*, 1–103. [CrossRef]
25. National Library of Medicine (US). Norethindrone. In *Drugs and Lactation Database (LactMed)*; National Library of Medicine (US): Bethesda, MD, USA, 2006.

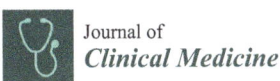

Review

Estetrol: A New Choice for Contraception

Franca Fruzzetti *,†, Tiziana Fidecicchi †, Maria Magdalena Montt Guevara and Tommaso Simoncini

Department of Obstetrics and Gynecology, Pisa University Hospital, 56126 Pisa, Italy; t.fidecicchi@gmail.com (T.F.); magdalena.montt@gmail.com (M.M.M.G.); tommaso.simoncini@unipi.it (T.S.)
* Correspondence: ffruzzi15@gmail.com; Tel.: +39-050-992-801
† Equally contributing authors.

Abstract: Estetrol (E4) is a natural estrogenic steroid that is normally produced by human fetal liver. Recent research has demonstrated that it is a potent, orally bioavailable, natural selective estrogen receptor modulator; it has a moderate affinity for both human estrogen receptor alpha (ERα) and ERβ, with a preference for ERα. Clinical studies have demonstrated possible use as an estrogen in combined oral contraceptives (COC). COCs containing E4 and drospirenone (DRSP) showed a high acceptability, tolerability, and user satisfaction also when compared to COCs containing ethinylestradiol (EE). E4/DRSP effectively inhibits ovulation, with a similar effect on endometrium thickness than that of EE-containing COCs. Low doses (15 mg) of E4 with DRSP (3 mg) showed promising results in term of bleeding pattern and cycle control, also when compared to other COCs containing synthetic estrogens. Moreover, the association has limited effects on serum lipids, liver, SHBG levels, and carbohydrate metabolism. This combination also could drive a lower risk of venous thromboembolism than EE-containing COCs. In this review, we will summarize the actual knowledge about the new E4-containing contraceptive. Further large-scale studies in the full target population are needed to provide more insights into the cardiovascular safety profile and user satisfaction of E4/DRSP.

Keywords: combined hormonal contraception; estetrol; metabolism; SHBG; cycle control; hemostasis

1. Introduction

Estetrol (E4) is a human natural estrogen which was discovered in 1965 in urines of pregnant women [1,2]. It is only produced during human pregnancy and it reaches the maternal circulation through the placenta [3,4]. Human maternal plasma levels increase during pregnancy, reaching high concentrations towards the end of gestation (≥1 ng/mL). Fetal plasma levels have been reported to be nearly 20 times higher than maternal plasma levels at parturition [5]. After delivery, blood levels of E4 become rapidly undetectable [6,7]. It is of interest that E4 is not produced by other species tested so far (mice, rat, and rabbit). The role as a marker of fetal health have been studied for many years but no correlation was found [7,8]. Even now the physiological significance of E4 in pregnancy is unknown.

In this review we summarize the actual knowledge about E4, focusing the attention on its new application for hormonal contraception.

2. Biosynthesis and Pharmacological Properties

Its chemical structure is the 15-hydroxyethryol or the oestra-1,3,5(10)-trien-3,15-16,17-tethrol: the molecule has 4-OH groups, so it's also called with the name E4 (Figure 1).

E4 is synthesized during pregnancy from estradiol (E2) and estriol (E3) by two fetal liver enzymes through hydroxylation. These two enzymes are *15α* and *16α-hydroxylase* and they are expressed only during fetal age [4].

E4 is extensively metabolized or inactivated by human hepatocytes in vitro, producing metabolites by direct glucuronidation of the D-ring and direct sulfation at an unconfirmed site. E4 is mainly excreted in the urine rather than through the biliary route, and it is the

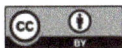

terminal product of its own pathway: there are not secondary reactions that could produce E3, E2, or estrone (E1) [9,10].

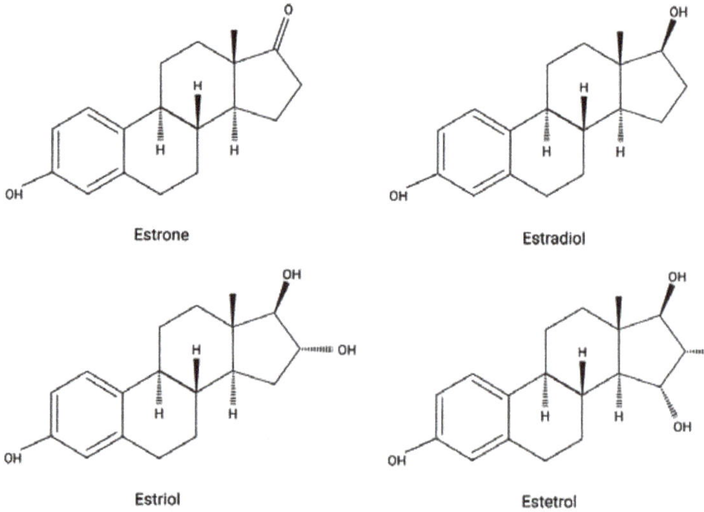

Figure 1. Molecular structure of different estrogens. Created with BioRender.com (4 September 2021).

E4 displays moderate protein binding (close to 50%) in human plasma. E4 does not bind to human sex hormone-binding globulin (SHBG) [11]. It is equally distributed between plasma and blood cells in human blood. E4 has a high oral bioavailability (90%) and an important long half-life in humans, with an average of 28–32 h half-life, which is about two-fold longer than E2 [9]. In contrast to E2, E4 does not show clinically relevant inhibiting or inducing interactions with cytochrome P450 liver enzymes or with other molecules [11,12].

In the 1970s and 1980s different studies demonstrated that E4 has a weaker estrogenic activity than E2, E3, and tamoxifen: this activity has been shown in uterus [5,7,8]. In fact, study shows that E4 has a low to moderate affinity for both human estrogen receptor α (ERα) and β (ERβ) with a 4/5-fold preference for ERα [10]. Based on this relatively low receptor binding affinity compared to E2, E4 was originally thought to be a weak estrogen [12,13].

Recent studies indicate that E4 is an estrogen with a distinctive profile of ERα activation. E4 activates the nuclear ERα, but it is an antagonist of the membrane ERα, in contrast to other estrogens [14–16]. Based on its pharmacological profile, E4 can be classified as the first Natural Estrogen with Selective Action in Tissues (NEST) [17]. NEST activities of E4 are the consequence of its unique dual role.

Effects on Different Tissues

E4 may display different effects on different tissues due to its agonist or antagonist activity on ERs.

In well validated and predictive rat models, E4 behaves as an estrogen agonist in all tissues investigated, i.e., bone, vagina, myometrium, endometrium, and brain, and it is effective in inhibiting ovulation by reducing follicle stimulating hormone (FSH) and luteinizing hormone (LH) plasma concentrations [8,18,19]. A study reported a beneficial effect of E4 on bone, through the analysis of different markers like: bone mineral density (BMD), mineralization of vertebral bodies from L3 to L5, strength against biomechanical damages and level of serum osteocalcin [18]. Another set of study was done on CNS, suggesting a neuroprotective role of E4 [19,20]. It was observed that in ovariectomized rats treated with E4 the expression of allopregnanolone and β-endorphin in serum was increased and different cerebral areas like frontal cortex, hippocampus, and pituitary gland were induced. The expression of those neurosteroids are reduced when E4 and E2 are given together [19,20].

Most beneficial effects of E4 on the vascular system have been ascribed to the activation of the membrane ERα of vascular endothelial cells, including enhancement of nitric oxide (NO) production, vasodilation, and prevention of atherosclerosis, of neointimal proliferation, and of hypertension [8].

On breast tumor tissue it acts as an estrogen antagonist in the presence of E2 [21,22]. The estrogen-antagonistic effect of E4 in the breast has been further supported by a recent pre-clinical study that has been performed in women with breast cancer, finding that E4 reduces breast cancer cells proliferation [21,23–26]. These features could suggest a future role of E4 as a selective estrogen receptor modulator (SERM), but with less adverse effect than tamoxifen (hot flushes, nausea, hypertension, thromboembolic events, endometrial hyperplasia) [24,27,28]. However, in 2008 a study showed that E4 has a weak proliferative activity on mammary tumoral MCF-7 cells [27] and surprisingly it acts as an estrogen antagonist on rat breast DMBA model cells, where it prevents the development of new breast tumors and stimulates the regression of pre-existing ones [28,29].

Some of the principal physiological role and properties of E4 on different tissues like bone, uterus, vagina, breast, CNS, and ovaries are shown in Table 1.

Table 1. Effects of estetrol on the estrogen receptor α (ERα) and β (ERβ) on different tissues: brain, bone, female genital system, and breast.

	Low affinity for estrogen receptors [12,13] Higher affinity for ERα than ERβ [10] A natural SERM [24,27,28]
	Neuroprotective effects [19,20] Inhibition of LH and FSH secretion [8,18,19]
	Prevention of bone demineralization [18] Increase bone mineral density [18]
	Inhibition of ovulation [30] Uterine growth and epithelial proliferation [16,31,32]
	Less known Estrogenic and anti-estrogenic effects on horizontal migration and matrix invasion of ER+ T47-D [19,30,33]

These features are very important because they mean that E4 could be a useful and safe molecule in hormonal therapy. In this field, an important application of E4 is for combined oral contraceptives (COCs). It holds promises for the safety and tolerability of COCs containing E4.

3. New Combined Hormonal Contraception with Estetrol

COCs traditionally contain an estrogen and a progestin component. Estrogens are useful to stabilize the endometrium, to regulate menstrual bleeding and to reduce follicle development. The most used estrogen is ethinylestradiol (EE), variously combined with different progestins, but it has an impact on liver function and endothelium that can produce rare cases of venous or arterial thrombotic complications. Since 2009 COCs containing E2 has been developed to reduce this effect. E4 may represent another valid option for COCs, with many advantages linked to its dual effect on receptors.

3.1. Ovulation and Cycle Control: How to Reach the Best Patients' Satisfaction

The ovulation inhibitory potency of E4 was first studied in preclinical models, followed by clinical trials in women (Table 2).

Coelingh Bennink et al. in 2008 [30] studied the effectiveness of E4 as an ovulation inhibitor in regularly cycling rats compared to EE. Rats were treated orally twice daily for four consecutive days with E4 (0.03, 0.1, 0.3, 1.0, or 3.0 mg/kg), EE (0.0003, 0.001, 0.003, 0.01, or 0.03 mg/kg) or vehicle control. Ovulation was significantly inhibited with a dose of 0.3 mg/kg of E4 twice daily and above and with 0.03 mg/kg of EE twice daily. In a second experiment they also administered 2.0 mg/kg of E4 once daily or divided in two doses of 1.0 mg/kg: this second option was able to inhibit ovulation in all treated rats, while the single-dose administration acted in half of them. EE resulted to be 18 times more potent than E4 [30].

The ability to suppress LH and FSH production in female humans was studied in early post-menopause women. E4 showed a profound central inhibitory and dose dependent effect on LH and FSH in post-menopause women [33]. After a single-dose administration, a clear dose-dependent inhibition of LH levels and a profound inhibition of FSH levels over 48 h after 100 mg of E4 (lasting over 7 days) was observed [9].

A phase II dose-finding pilot study evaluated the efficacy of different dosages of E4 combined with levonorgestrel (LNG) or drospirenone (DRSP) in suppressing the pituitary-ovarian axis and ovulation in healthy premenopausal women [31]. E4 combined with DRSP (5 or 10 mg E4 + 3 mg DRSP) or LNG (5, 10 or 20 mg E4 + 0.15 mg LNG) in a 24/4-day regimen was compared to EE 20 mcg + 3 mg DRSP, all of them administered for three consecutive cycles. The highest suppression of ovarian activity was observed in the 20 mg E4/LNG group and was very similar to that observed with EE/DRSP. However, there were no ovulations during the treatment cycles in all treatment groups, showing the efficacy of all the combinations of E4. Endometrial thickness was also reduced similarly during treatment in all treatment groups.

The first post-treatment ovulation occurred approximately 17 days after the last treatment day in the E4/DRSP groups, and 21 days after the last active treatment in the E4/LNG and EE/DRSP groups: this period was comparable to the duration of a normal follicular phase, confirming adequate ovarian suppression during treatment. In conclusion, a dosage above 10 mg/day of E4 with DRSP or LNG demonstrated to be a promising combination for contraception [31].

Table 2. Phase II and phase III studies about new estetrol (E4)-containing combined oral contraceptives (COCs) are summarized. Studies are divided according to the outcomes studied.

Outcomes.	Study	E4 Combinations Tested	Comparators	Results
Ovulation inhibition and cycle control	Phase II Duijkers et al., 2015 [31]	5 or 10 mg E4 + 3 mg DRSP 5, 10, or 20 mg E4 + 0.15 mg LNG 24 + 4 regimen	0.02 mg EE + 3 mg DRSP 24 + 4 regimen	No ovulation in any treatment group. Ovarian activity inhibition proportional to E4 dosage (20 mg E4/LNG like EE/DRSP) Endometrial thickness similarly suppressed in all groups Post-treatment ovulation occurred in all patients in the first month.
	Phase II Apter et al., 2016 [32]	15 or 20 mg E4 + 3 mg DRSP 15 or 20 mg E4 + 0.15 mg LNG 24 + 4 regimen	4-phasic commercial packaging of E2V/DNG 26 + 2 regimen	Lowest frequency of unscheduled bleeding and/or spotting and absence of withdrawal bleeding in the 15 mg E4/DRSP group
	Phase III Gemzell-Danielsson et al., 2021 [34]	15 mg E4 + 3 mg DRSP 24 + 4 regimen	/	Method-failure PI: 0.29 pregnancies/100 woman-years Scheduled bleeding occurred in 91.9–94.4% of women per cycle Unscheduled bleeding/spotting episodes decreased in the first 6 cycles and remained stable thereafter (<16%)
	Phase III Creinin et al., 2021 [35]	15 mg E4 + 3 mg DRSP 24 + 4 regimen	/	Method-failure PI in 16–35 years old women: 1.43 pregnancies/100 woman-years Scheduled bleeding occurred in 82.9 to 87.0% of women per cycle Unscheduled bleeding decreased in the first 4 cycles and remained stable thereafter (15.5% to 19.2%)
Treatment satisfaction	Phase II Apter et al., 2017 [36]	15 or 20 mg E4 + 3 mg DRSP 15 or 20 mg E4 + 0.15 mg LNG 24 + 4 regimen	4-phasic commercial packaging of E2V/DNG 26 + 2 regimen	The largest proportion of treatment satisfaction in the 15 mg E4/DRSP group; the lowest in the 15 mg/LNG group Well-being with E4/DRSP: better than with E4/LNG Proportion of women with a 2 kg or more weight loss: the highest with 15 mg E4/DRSP
Hemostatic effect	Phase II Kluft et al., 2017 [37]	5 or 10 mg E4 + 3 mg DRSP 24 + 4 regimen	0.02 mg EE + 3 mg DRSP 24 + 4 regimen	E4/DRSP no or minor effect on markers of coagulation inhibition; they were reduced by EE/DRSP thus promoting coagulation E4/DRSP did not increase D-dimer levels, unlike EE/DRSP
	Phase II Douxfils et al., 2020 [38]	15 mg E4 + 3 mg DRSP 24 + 4 regimen	0.02 mg EE + 3 mg DRSP 24 + 4 regimen 0.03 mg EE + 0.15 mg LNG 21 + 7 regimen	Changes in hemostasis parameters after treatment with 6 cycles of E4/DRSP were smaller or like those observed for EE/LNG Similar, but more pronounced changes were also observed versus EE/DRSP

Table 2. Cont.

Outcomes	Study	E4 Combinations Tested	Comparators	Results
Metabolic effect	Phase II Mawet et al., 2015 [39]	5 or 10 mg E4 + 3 mg DRSP 5, 10, or 20 mg E4 + 0.15 mg LNG 24 + 4 regimen	0.02 mg EE + 3 mg DRSP 24 + 4 regimen	Minor effects on lipid levels (HDL- and LDL- cholesterol) with E4/DRSP and E4/LNG Triglycerides levels: reduced with E4/LNG, the same with E4/DRSP and increased with EE/DRSP
	Phase II Klipping et al., 2021 [40]	15 mg E4 + 3 mg DRSP 24 + 4 regimen	0.03 mg EE + 0.15 mg LNG 21 + 7 regimen 0.02 mg EE + 3 mg DRSP 24 + 4 regimen	E4/DRSP had minimal impact on lipid parameters The largest effect was observed for triglycerides, still less than EE/LNG and EE/DRSP E4/DRSP: no effect on carbohydrate metabolism
SHBG and other liver proteins	Phase II Klipping et al., 2021 [40]	15 mg E4 + 3 mg DRSP 24 + 4 regimen	0.03 mg EE + 0.15 mg LNG 21 + 7 regimen 0.02 mg EE + 3 mg DRSP 24 + 4 regimen	Liver proteins, except CRP, increased in all groups, but the effect for angiotensinogen and SHBG was less pronunced with E4/DRSP compared to EE/LNG and EE/DRSP
	Phase II Mawet et al., 2015 [39]	5 or 10 mg E4 + 3 mg DRSP 5, 10, or 20 mg E4 + 0.15 mg LNG 24 + 4 regimen	0.02 mg EE + 3 mg DRSP 24 + 4 regimen	SHBG and other liver proteins were minimally or not affected by E4/LNG and E4/DRSP Changes of SHBG and other liver proteins were more marked in the EE/DRSP group
	Phase II Kluft et al., 2017 [37]	5 or 10 mg E4 + 3 mg DRSP 24 + 4 regimen	0.02 mg EE + 3 mg DRSP 24 + 4 regimen	SHBG and angiotensinogen increase with 10 mg E4/DRSP was 15%–20% that of EE/DRSP 5 or 10 mg E4/DRSP had nearly no effect on SHBG and minor effect on angiotensinogen
	Phase II Douxfils et al., 2020 [38]	15 mg E4 + 3 mg DRSP 24 + 4 regimen	0.02 mg EE + 3 mg DRSP 24 + 4 regimen 0.03 mg EE + 0.15 mg LNG 21 + 7 regimen	Changes in SHBG values for E4/DRSP, EE/LNG and EE/DRSP were +55%, +74% and +251%, respectively
Bones: safety study	Phase II Mawet et al., 2015 [39]	5 or 10 mg E4 + 3 mg DRSP 5, 10, or 20 mg E4 + 0.15 mg LNG 24 + 4 regimen	0.02 mg EE + 3 mg DRSP 24 + 4 regimen	E4 groups: dose-related decrease of biomarkers of bone resorption (C-telopeptide) and bone formation (osteocalcin) Decreased bone turnover in all E4 and EE combinations: it is indicative of a similar positive influence on bone turnover in young post-adolescent women

CRP, C-reactive protein; DNG, dienogest; DRSP, drospirenone; E2V, estradiol valerate; EE, ethinylestradiol; HDL, high density lipoprotein; LDL, low density lipoprotein; LNG, levonorgestrel; PI, pearl index; SHBG, sex hormone binding globulin.

Another phase II study aimed to assess bleeding patterns and cycle control of E4 containing COCs in a 24/4-day regimen, using a COC containing estradiol valerate (E2V) and dienogest (DNG) as a reference [32]. E4 15 and 20 mg/DRSP 3 mg, E4 20 mg/LNG 0.15 mg and E2V/DNG were compared after six treatment cycles. The frequency of unscheduled bleeding/spotting was lower in the E4/DRSP groups compared to the other treatment groups: by cycle 6, the frequency varied between 33.8% in the group using 15 mg of E4 + DRSP and 47.8% in the E2V/DNG group, with increasing intensity of unscheduled bleeding over time in the E2V/DNG group. For E4/DRSP, the frequency of absence of withdrawal bleeding was 3.5 (15 mg E4) to 3.8% (20 mg E4) at cycle 6. In the E4/LNG groups, the frequencies were 14.0–18.5%, and for E2V/DNG it was 27.1%. Only 8.9% of subjects in the group using 15 mg of E4 + DRSP discontinued prematurely. In conclusion, the 15 mg E4/DRSP combination has been shown to be the most efficacious in terms of bleeding pattern and cycle control, compared with the other combinations investigated [32]. The largest proportion of treatment satisfaction was reported for 15 mg E4/DRSP (73.1%) compared to 20 mg E4/DRSP and 15 or 20 mg E4/LNG. Well-being with E4/DRSP combinations was statistically significantly better than with E4/LNG combinations and the administration of 15 mg E4/DRSP favors a good weight control, with 36.7% of women losing 2 kg or more after 6 months of treatment [36].

After these dose-finding studies, phase III clinical trials using the combination E4 15 mg/DRSP 3 mg were performed. Two studies are available by now, for a total of around 3400 women enrolled and followed for a period of 13 cycles. In the first study conducted in 1864 women aged 16 to 50 years old from North America, the PI was 2.65 in women aged 16 to 35 (54% of the undesired pregnancies due to method failure, with a method-failure PI of 1.43) [35]. In the second study, conducted in 1553 women from Europe and Russia between the ages of 18 and 50 years old, less pregnancies were reported, and the Pearl Index (PI) was 0.47 in the group aged 18 to 35 and 0.41 in the whole group, with a method-failure PI of 0.25 in the whole group. This was considered a sufficiently low value for an oral contraceptive. Scheduled bleeding occurred in 91.9–94.4% of participants per cycle. Scheduled bleeding and/or spotting days remained stable throughout the study with a median duration of 4 to 5 days. Unscheduled bleeding and/or spotting episodes after Cycle 1 occurred in 19.2% of women in Cycle 2 and decreased to 12.8% of women in Cycle 11. Among these episodes over all cycles, 71.8% were spotting-only episodes, 22.7% were mixed bleeding/spotting and 5.4% were bleeding-only [34]. Overall, a COC with E4 15 mg/DRSP 3 mg was considered effective at preventing unwanted pregnancies with a satisfactory bleeding pattern control.

3.2. Hemostatic effect

Historically, EE containing COCs demonstrated their efficacy and safety, with a satisfactory bleeding pattern. However, their impact on liver function and vascular endothelium could produce rare cardiovascular thrombotic complications that could limit their use in a subgroup of women. The use of androgenic progestins and the substitution of EE with E2 can modulate and reduce this risk [41,42]. E4 represents a promising option to be used for COCs. From in vitro to in vivo studies investigated its influence on hemostatic parameters.

In an in vitro study on human umbilical vein endothelial cells, the effects of E4 on fibrinolytic system and whether it could influence the ability of endothelial cells to migrate were studied [43]. Expression of plasminogen-activator inhibitor-1 (PAI-1), urokinase-type plasminogen activator (u-PA), and tissue plasminogen activator (t-PA) proteins were all increased by E4 in a dose-dependent manner, although E4 was less effective than equimolar amounts of E2. Moreover, endothelial cell migration capacity was increased by E4 treatment. So, it was concluded that E4 could regulate the fibrinolytic protein system in endothelial cells, with potential implications for the local control of blood clotting and for vascular remodeling [43].

Mouse models were also used to test E4 impact on arterial and venous thrombosis. It increased mouse tail bleeding time, it protected from both arterial and venous thrombosis, and it induced a resistance against acute thromboembolism. Ex vivo flow-based adhesion studies conducted in whole blood under arterial flow conditions on a collagen matrix showed that E4 treatment also reduced platelet adhesion [15].

In human studies using the new COC containing E4, more insights about this issue were given (Table 2). Kluft et al. [37] evaluated the effects of 3 mg DRSP in combination with 5 or 10 mg of E4 compared to a preparation containing EE 20 µg/DRSP 3 mg. Over three months, the E4-containing preparations had a much lower impact. Both E4 combinations reduced D-dimer level with no effect on antithrombin, protein S activity or activated protein C resistance, and the 5 mg E4/DRSP combination also decreased prothrombin fragment 1 + 2. It can be stated that E4/DRSP have a considerably lower hepatic and vascular estrogenicity than EE/DRSP [37].

In addition, Douxfils et al. [38] demonstrated that after six months of treatment E4 15 mg/DRSP 3 mg caused similar or smaller changes in procoagulant, anticoagulant, and fibrinolytic parameters than EE/LNG, while the difference with EE/DRSP was more pronounced [38].

3.3. Estetrol, Metabolism, and Cardiovascular Risk

One of the earliest manifestations of atherosclerosis is the dysfunction of the vascular endothelium, caused by one or more "insults" to the endothelium. This leads to a decrease in release of the vasodilator, nitric oxide, and an increase in production of the vasoconstrictor, endothelin-1. Although endothelial dysfunction occurs early in the atherosclerotic process, it continues throughout the progression of the disease. A second major consequence of damage to the endothelium is the accumulation of inflammatory cells in the vascular wall, that causes the oxidation and accumulation of low-density lipoproteins (LDL). This activates a vicious cycle which leads to the atheroma [44].

Estrogens are known to have a vasculoprotective action, which has been demonstrated clearly in animal models of early atheroma: E2 has been shown to strongly prevent fatty streak deposition in monkeys, rabbits, and mice [45]. They have a general cardioprotective effect: they prevent atherosclerosis [46,47], they reduce hypertensive effects of ovariectomy [48], they reduce age- and hypertension-related arterial stiffening [49], they increase the production of nitric oxide [50], they accelerate endothelial reparation processes [51], they prevent intimal post-traumatic hyperplasia [52].

E4 demonstrated to have similar vasculoprotective action in mice thanks to its binding with ERα, even if with less potence than E2 [53–55]. Moreover, it has positive effects on metabolic parameters. A study in post-menopausal women treated with different doses of E4 (2 mg, 10 mg, 20 mg, or 40 mg) for 28 days showed that a lowering effect on LDL was accompanied with an increase in HDL and no or minimal changes in triglycerides; all the effects were dose-dependent [56].

E4 associations with different progestins were studied to evaluate their metabolic effects, in view of the formulation of new COCs (Table 2). Mawet et al. [39] made a dose-finding study in healthy normally ovulating women aged 18–35 years. They administered six different treatments in six groups of women for three consecutive cycles in a 24/4-day regimen: 5 mg or 10 mg of E4 with 3 mg of DRSP; 5 mg, 10 mg, or 20 mg E4 with 0.15 mg LNG; 0.02 mg EE with 3 mg DRSP as comparator. E4-containing COCs caused minor effects on lipoproteins and triglycerides compared to the EE/DRSP group [39]. In addition Klipping et al. [40] found similar results. The combination of 15 mg of E4 and 3 mg of DRSP had minimal impact on lipid parameters. The largest effect was observed for triglycerides, that showed a 24% increase after treatment; however, this increase was less compared to EE/LNG (+28%) and EE/DRSP (+65.5%) [40].

Phase III studies will better address this issue, giving information on a large population. However, phase II results show that E4/DRSP combination is substantially neutral on lipid parameters.

3.4. Effects on the Synthesis of Other Liver Proteins

E4-containing COCs have a limited effect on liver function (Table 2).

SHBG is a carrier protein produced in the liver. It binds estrogens and testosterone, and its levels may be used as a surrogate to evaluate the steroid effects on the liver. SHBG may be considered as a marker for estrogenicity of a contraceptive preparation and possibly for the risk of venous thrombosis [57,58]. In general, estrogens can cause a dose-related increase of SHBG levels, while progestogens induce a decrease of SHBG levels, depending on the type and the dose of the progestogen used. Thus, the combination of the estrogenic effect of the estrogen contained in the hormonal contraceptive and of the antiestrogenic effect of the progestogen used (effect that is higher with androgenic progestins) determines the total estrogenicity of that hormonal contraceptive.

SHBG plasma levels decreased with E4 (5, 10, or 20 mg)/LNG, while showed a dose-dependent slight increase with 5 or 10 mg E4/DRSP (+7.9–44.5%). This increase is considerably less than with EE/DRSP [39]. In addition Klipping et al. [40] found a similar variation of SHBG: E4 15 mg/DRSP 3 mg caused an increase of 87.15% of SHBG levels at cycle 6, still less than EE/LNG and EE/DRSP [40]. Other studies confirmed the little influence of this COC on SHBG production [37,38]. Other liver proteins were studied, too. Angiotensinogen changes showed a profile similar to SHBG [45,46,59]. C-reactive protein, cortisol binding globulin, thyroxin binding globulin, and ceruloplasmin showed slight changes with E4/DRSP [39,40], confirming the limited estrogenic effect of E4 on liver also when combined to antiandrogenic progestins.

3.5. Bones and Breast: Safety of E4-Containing COCs

Studies about the effects of the new proposed COCs with E4 on tissues like bone and breast are still scant.

Even if some data about the preventive effect on bone loss of E4 alone are already available [18,59], by now the only available information about effects on bone of E4-containing COCs is given by the study by Mawet et al. [39] (Table 2). A balance between bone resorption and bone formation maintains the regulation of bone mineral density. This study did not detect any imbalances after treatment with E4/DRSP, E4/LNG or the comparator EE/DRSP in serum osteocalcin (a marker of bone formation) and C-telopeptide (a marker of bone degradation). This may be indicative of a positive influence on bone turnover in young post-adolescent women, similarly to EE- or E2-containing COCs [39].

Similarly, very little is known about the effects of E4/DRSP combinations on breast. Recently, a study on breast cancer was published [60]. It shows that E4 combined with or without progesterone or DRSP promotes neither breast cancer development nor metastatic dissemination in three different models of breast cancer when used at a therapeutic dose for hormone replacement therapy or COC [60]. The results may suggest that the use of E4 in contraception could further limit the already minimal possible effect of other hormonal contraceptives on breast cancer risk. Nevertheless, at the present it is not possible to extrapolate clinical data about this issue.

4. Conclusions

In conclusion, pharmacological properties of E4 make it a useful molecule for hormonal therapies and contraception. By now, some phase II and phase III studies gave promising results using the combination of E4 15 mg/DRSP 3 mg: this COCs showed a good contraceptive effect and cycle control, with a neutral metabolic effect. However, still very little is known about the effects of this new combination on breast and bone. Post-marketing studies are needed to consolidate the available data and to explore all the possible side effects and risks for bone, breast, and cardiovascular system of a long-term use of E4-containing pills compared to the well-known EE- and E2-containing combinations.

Author Contributions: All authors have substantially contributed to the work. All authors have read and agreed to the published version of the manuscript.

Funding: Authors received no external funding.

Conflicts of Interest: The authors declare no conflict of interest.

References

1. Hagen, A.; Barr, M. Metabolism of 17β-oestradiol-4-14C in early infancy. *Endocrinology* **1965**, *49*, 207–220. [CrossRef]
2. Zucconi, G.; Lisboa, B.P.; Simonitsch, E.; Roth, L.; Hagen, A.A.; Diczfalusy, E. Isolation of 15-alpha-hydroxy-oestriol from pregnancy urine and from the urine of newborn infants. *Acta Endocrinol.* **1967**, *56*, 413–423. [CrossRef] [PubMed]
3. Schwers, J.; Eriksson, G.; Wiqvist, N.; Diczfalusy, E. 15α-hydroxylation: A new pathway of estrogen metabolism in the human fetus and newborn. *BBA—Gen. Subj.* **1965**, *100*, 313–316. [CrossRef]
4. Schwers, J.; Eriksson, G.; Diczfalusy, E. Metabolism of oestrone and oestradiol in the human foeto-placental unit at midpregnancy. *Acta Endocrinol.* **1965**, *49*, 65–82. [CrossRef]
5. Coelingh Bennink, F.; Holinka, C.F.; Visser, M.; Coelingh Bennink, H.J.T. Maternal and fetal estetrol levels during pregnancy. *Climacteric* **2008**, *11*, 69–72. [CrossRef]
6. Tulchinsky, D.; Frigoletto, F.D.; Ryan, K.J.; Fishman, J. Plasma estetrol as an index of fetal well-being. *Obstet. Gynecol. Surv.* **1976**, *31*, 9–10. [CrossRef]
7. Kundu, N.; Wachs, M.; Iverson, G.B.; Petersen, L.P. Comparison of serum unconjugated estriol and estetrol in normal and complicated pregnancies. *Obstet. Gynecol.* **1981**, *58*, 276–281.
8. Visser, M.; Coelingh Bennink, H.J.T. Clinical applications for estetrol. *J. Steroid Biochem. Mol. Biol.* **2009**, *114*, 85–89. [CrossRef]
9. Visser, M.; Holinka, C.F.; Coelingh Bennink, H.J.T.T. First human exposure to exogenous single-dose oral estetrol in early postmenopausal women. *Climacteric* **2008**, *11*, 31–40. [CrossRef] [PubMed]
10. Visser, M.; Foidart, J.M.; Coelingh Bennink, H.J.T. In vitro effects of estetrol on receptor binding, drug targets and human liver cell metabolism. *Climacteric* **2008**, *11*, 64–68. [CrossRef] [PubMed]
11. Hammond, G.L.; Hogeveen, K.N.; Visser, M.; Coelingh Bennink, H.J.T. Estetrol does not bind sex hormone binding globulin or increase its production by human HepG2 cells. *Climacteric* **2008**, *11*, 41–46. [CrossRef]
12. Coelingh Bennink, H.J.T.; Holinka, C.F.; Diczfalusy, E. Estetrol review: Profile and potential clinical applications. *Climacteric* **2008**, *11*, 47–58. [CrossRef]
13. Holinka, C.F.; Brincat, M.; Coelingh Bennink, H.J.T. Preventive effect of oral estetrol in a menopausal hot flush model. *Climacteric* **2008**, *11*, 15–21. [CrossRef]
14. Abot, A.; Fontaine, C.; Buscato, M.; Solinhac, R.; Flouriot, G.; Fabre, A.; Drougard, A.; Rajan, S.; Laine, M.; Milon, A.; et al. The uterine and vascular actions of estetrol delineate a distinctive profile of estrogen receptor α modulation, uncoupling nuclear and membrane activation. *EMBO Mol. Med.* **2014**, *6*, 1328–1346. [CrossRef] [PubMed]
15. Valéra, M.C.; Noirrit-Esclassan, E.; Dupuis, M.; Fontaine, C.; Lenfant, F.; Briaux, A.; Cabou, C.; Garcia, C.; Lairez, O.; Foidart, J.M.; et al. Effect of estetrol, a selective nuclear estrogen receptor modulator, in mouse models of arterial and venous thrombosis. *Mol. Cell. Endocrinol.* **2018**, *477*, 132–139. [CrossRef]
16. Benoit, T.; Valera, M.C.; Fontaine, C.; Buscato, M.; Lenfant, F.; Raymond-Letron, I.; Tremollieres, F.; Soulie, M.; Foidart, J.M.; Game, X.; et al. Estetrol, a Fetal Selective Estrogen Receptor Modulator, Acts on the Vagina of Mice through Nuclear Estrogen Receptor α Activation. *Am. J. Pathol.* **2017**, *187*, 2499–2507. [CrossRef]
17. Foidart, J.M.; Gaspard, U.; Pequeux, C.; Jost, M.; Gordenne, V.; Tskitishvili, E.; Gallez, A.; Valera, M.C.; Gourdy, P.; Fontaine, C.; et al. Unique Vascular Benefits of Estetrol, a Native Fetal Estrogen with Specific Actions in Tissues (NEST). In *Sex Steroids' Effects on Brain, Heart and Vessels*; Springer: Cham, Switzerland, 2019; pp. 169–195. [CrossRef]
18. Coelingh Bennink, H.J.T.; Heegaard, A.M.; Visser, M.; Holinka, C.F.; Christiansen, C. Oral bioavailability and bone-sparing effects of estetrol in an osteoporosis model. *Climacteric* **2008**, *11*, 2–14. [CrossRef] [PubMed]
19. Pluchino, N.; Drakopoulos, P.; Casarosa, E.; Freschi, L.; Petignat, P.; Yaron, M.; Genazzani, A.R. Effect of estetrol on beta-endorphin level in female rats. *Steroids* **2015**, *95*, 104–110. [CrossRef] [PubMed]
20. Pluchino, N.; Santoro, A.N.; Casarosa, E.; Giannini, A.; Genazzani, A.; Russo, M.; Russo, N.; Petignat, P.; Genazzani, A.R. Effect of estetrol administration on brain and serum allopregnanolone in intact and ovariectomized rats. *J. Steroid Biochem. Mol. Biol.* **2014**, *143*, 285–290. [CrossRef]
21. Giretti, M.S.M.S.; Montt Guevara, M.M.; Cecchi, E.; Mannella, P.; Palla, G.; Spina, S.; Bernacchi, G.; Di Bello, S.; Genazzani, A.R.; Genazzani, A.D.; et al. Effects of Estetrol on Migration and Invasion in T47-D Breast Cancer Cells through the Actin Cytoskeleton. *Front. Endocrinol.* **2014**, *5*, 1–9. [CrossRef]
22. Gérard, C.; Blacher, S.; Communal, L.; Courtin, A.; Tskitishvili, E.; Mestdagt, M.; Munaut, C.; Noel, A.; Gompel, A.; Péqueux, C.; et al. Estetrol is a weak estrogen antagonizing estradiol-dependent mammary gland proliferation. *J. Endocrinol.* **2014**, *224*, 85–95. [CrossRef] [PubMed]
23. Singer, C.F.; Bennink, H.J.T.C.; Natter, C.; Steurer, S.; Rudas, M.; Moinfar, F.; Appels, N.; Visser, M.; Kubista, E. Antiestrogenic effects of the fetal estrogen estetrol in women with estrogen-receptor positive early breast cancer. *Carcinogenesis* **2014**, *35*, 2447–2451. [CrossRef]
24. Schmidt, M.; Lenhard, H.; Hoenig, A.; Zimmerman, Y.; Krijgh, J.; Jansen, M.; Coelingh Bennink, H.J.T. Tumor suppression, dose-limiting toxicity and wellbeing with the fetal estrogen estetrol in patients with advanced breast cancer. *J. Cancer Res. Clin. Oncol.* **2021**, *147*, 1833–1842. [CrossRef] [PubMed]

25. Gallez, A.; Dias Da Silva, I.; Wuidar, V.; Foidart, J.-M.; Péqueux, C. Estetrol and Mammary Gland: Friends or Foes? *J. Mammary Gland Biol. Neoplasia* **2021**. [CrossRef]
26. Liu, S.; Ruan, X.; Schultz, S.; Neubauer, H.; Fehm, T.; Seeger, H.; Mueck, A.O. Oestetrol stimulates proliferation and oestrogen receptor expression in breast cancer cell lines: Comparison of four oestrogens. *Eur. J. Contracept. Reprod. Health Care* **2015**, *20*, 29–35. [CrossRef]
27. Jozan, S.; Kreitmann, B.; Bayard, F. Different effects of oestradiol, oestriol, oestetrol and of oestrone on human breast cancer cells (MCF-7) in long term tissue culture. *Acta Endocrinol.* **1981**, *98*, 73–80. [CrossRef] [PubMed]
28. Coelingh Bennink, H.J.T.; Singer, C.; Simoncini, T.; Genazzani, A.R.; Holinka, C.F.; Kubista, E. Estetrol, a pregnancy-specific human steroid, prevents and suppresses mammary tumor growth in a rat model. *Climacteric* **2008**, *11*, 29. [CrossRef]
29. Visser, M.; Kloosterboer, H.J.J.; Bennink, H.J.T.C.; Coelingh Bennink, H.J.T.; Kloosterboer, H.J.J. Estetrol prevents and suppresses mammary tumors induced by DMBA in a rat model. *Horm. Mol. Biol. Clin. Investig.* **2012**, *9*, 95–103. [CrossRef]
30. Coelingh Bennink, H.J.T.; Skouby, S.; Bouchard, P.; Holinka, C.F. Ovulation inhibition by estetrol in an in vivo model. *Contraception* **2008**, *77*, 186–190. [CrossRef]
31. Duijkers, I.J.M.; Klipping, C.; Zimmerman, Y.; Appels, N.; Jost, M.; Maillard, C.; Mawet, M.; Foidart, J.M.; Bennink, H.J.T.C. Inhibition of ovulation by administration of estetrol in combination with drospirenone or levonorgestrel: Results of a phase II dose-finding pilot study. *Eur. J. Contracept. Reprod. Health Care* **2015**, *20*, 476–489. [CrossRef]
32. Apter, D.; Zimmerman, Y.; Beekman, L.; Mawet, M.; Maillard, C.; Foidart, J.M.; Coelingh Bennink, H.J.T. Bleeding pattern and cycle control with estetrol-containing combined oral contraceptives: Results from a phase II, randomised, dose-finding study (FIESTA). *Contraception* **2016**, *94*, 366–373. [CrossRef] [PubMed]
33. Visser, M.; Coelingh Bennink, H.J.T. Estetrol, the new natural estrogen for clinical use in women. *Ref. Gynecol. Obstet.* **2011**, *14*, 427–432.
34. Gemzell-Danielsson, K.; Apter, D.; Zatik, J.; Weyers, S.; Piltonen, T.; Suturina, L.; Apolikhina, I.; Jost, M.; Creinin, M.D.; Foidart, J. Estetrol-Drospirenone combination oral contraceptive: A clinical study of contraceptive efficacy, bleeding pattern, and safety in Europe and Russia. *BJOG Int. J. Obstet. Gynaecol.* **2021**, 1–9. [CrossRef]
35. Creinin, M.D.; Westhoff, C.L.; Bouchard, C.; Chen, M.J.; Jensen, J.T.; Kaunitz, A.M.; Achilles, S.L.; Foidart, J.M.; Archer, D.F. Estetrol-drospirenone combination oral contraceptive: North American phase 3 efficacy and safety results. *Contraception* **2021**, *104*, 222–228. [CrossRef]
36. Apter, D.; Zimmerman, Y.; Beekman, L.; Mawet, M.; Maillard, C.; Foidart, J.M.; Coelingh Bennink, H.J.T. Estetrol combined with drospirenone: An oral contraceptive with high acceptability, user satisfaction, well-being and favourable body weight control. *Eur. J. Contracept. Reprod. Health Care* **2017**, *22*, 260–267. [CrossRef]
37. Kluft, C.; Zimmerman, Y.; Mawet, M.; Klipping, C.; Duijkers, I.J.M.; Neuteboom, J.; Foidart, J.M.; Bennink, H.C. Reduced hemostatic effects with drospirenone-based oral contraceptives containing estetrol vs. ethinyl estradiol. *Contraception* **2017**, *95*, 140–147. [CrossRef]
38. Douxfils, J.; Klipping, C.; Duijkers, I.; Kinet, V.; Mawet, M.; Maillard, C.; Jost, M.; Rosing, J.; Foidart, J.-M. Evaluation of the effect of a new oral contraceptive containing estetrol and drospirenone on hemostasis parameters. *Contraception* **2020**, *102*, 396–402. [CrossRef]
39. Mawet, M.; Maillard, C.; Klipping, C.; Zimmerman, Y.; Foidart, J.M.; Bennink, H.J.T.C. Unique effects on hepatic function, lipid metabolism, bone and growth endocrine parameters of estetrol in combined oral contraceptives. *Eur. J. Contracept. Reprod. Health Care* **2015**, *20*, 463–475. [CrossRef] [PubMed]
40. Klipping, C.; Duijkers, I.; Mawet, M.; Maillard, C.; Bastidas, A.; Jost, M.; Foidart, J.M. Endocrine and metabolic effects of an oral contraceptive containing estetrol and drospirenone. *Contraception* **2021**, *103*, 213–221. [CrossRef]
41. Stegeman, B.H.; de Bastos, M.; Rosendaal, F.R.; van Hylckama Vlieg, A.; Helmerhorst, F.M.; Stijnen, T.; Dekkers, O.M. Different combined oral contraceptives and the risk of venous thrombosis: Systematic review and network meta-analysis. *BMJ* **2013**, *347*, f5298. [CrossRef] [PubMed]
42. Farris, M.; Bastianelli, C.; Rosato, E.; Brosens, I.; Benagiano, G. Pharmacodynamics of combined estrogen-progestin oral contraceptives: 2. effects on hemostasis. *Expert Rev. Clin. Pharmacol.* **2017**, *10*, 1129–1144. [CrossRef]
43. Montt-Guevara, M.M.; Palla, G.; Spina, S.; Bernacchi, G.; Cecchi, E.; Campelo, A.E.; Shortrede, J.E.; Canu, A.; Simoncini, T. Regulatory effects of estetrol on the endothelial plasminogen pathway and endothelial cell migration. *Maturitas* **2017**, *99*, 1–9. [CrossRef] [PubMed]
44. Rahman, M.S.; Woollard, K. Atherosclerosis. *Adv. Exp. Med. Biol.* **2017**, *1003*, 121–144. [PubMed]
45. Arnal, J.-F.; Scarabin, P.-Y.; Trémollières, F.; Laurell, H.; Gourdy, P. Estrogens in vascular biology and disease: Where do we stand today? *Curr. Opin. Lipidol.* **2007**, *18*, 554–560. [CrossRef] [PubMed]
46. Hodgin, J.B.; Krege, J.H.; Reddick, R.L.; Korach, K.S.; Smithies, O.; Maeda, N. Estrogen receptor α is a major mediator of 17β-estradiol's atheroprotective effects on lesion size in Apoe−/− mice. *J. Clin. Investig.* **2001**, *107*, 333–340. [CrossRef]
47. Billon-Galés, A.; Fontaine, C.; Douin-Echinard, V.; Delpy, L.; Berges, H.; Calippe, B.; Lenfant, F.; Laurell, H.; Guéry, J.-C.; Gourdy, P.; et al. Endothelial Estrogen Receptor-α Plays a Crucial Role in the Atheroprotective Action of 17β-Estradiol in Low-Density Lipoprotein Receptor–Deficient Mice. *Circulation* **2009**, *120*, 2567–2576. [CrossRef]

48. Pollow, D.P.; Romero-Aleshire, M.J.; Sanchez, J.N.; Konhilas, J.P.; Brooks, H.L. ANG II-induced hypertension in the VCD mouse model of menopause is prevented by estrogen replacement during perimenopause. *Am. J. Physiol. Integr. Comp. Physiol.* **2015**, *309*, R1546–R1552. [CrossRef]
49. Tarhouni, K.; Freidja, M.L.; Guihot, A.L.; Vessieres, E.; Grimaud, L.; Toutain, B.; Lenfant, F.; Arnal, J.F.; Loufrani, L.; Henrion, D. Role of estrogens and age in flow-mediated outward remodeling of rat mesenteric resistance arteries. *Am. J. Physiol. Circ. Physiol.* **2014**, *307*, H504–H514. [CrossRef]
50. Darblade, B.; Pendaries, C.; Krust, A.; Dupont, S.; Fouque, M.-J.; Rami, J.; Chambon, P.; Bayard, F.; Arnal, J.-F. Estradiol Alters Nitric Oxide Production in the Mouse Aorta Through the α-, but not β-, Estrogen Receptor. *Circ. Res.* **2002**, *90*, 413–419. [CrossRef]
51. Brouchet, L.; Krust, A.; Dupont, S.; Chambon, P.; Bayard, F.; Arnal, J.F. Estradiol Accelerates Reendothelialization in Mouse Carotid Artery Through Estrogen Receptor-α but Not Estrogen Receptor-β. *Circulation* **2001**, *103*, 423–428. [CrossRef]
52. Smirnova, N.F.; Fontaine, C.; Buscato, M.; Lupieri, A.; Vinel, A.; Valera, M.-C.; Guillaume, M.; Malet, N.; Foidart, J.-M.; Raymond-Letron, I.; et al. The Activation Function-1 of Estrogen Receptor Alpha Prevents Arterial Neointima Development Through a Direct Effect on Smooth Muscle Cells. *Circ. Res.* **2015**, *117*, 770–778. [CrossRef]
53. Guivarc'h, E.; Buscato, M.; Guihot, A.L.; Favre, J.; Vessières, E.; Grimaud, L.; Wakim, J.; Melhem, N.J.; Zahreddine, R.; Adlanmerini, M.; et al. Predominant role of nuclear versus membrane estrogen receptor α in arterial protection: Implications for estrogen receptor α modulation in cardiovascular prevention/safety. *J. Am. Heart Assoc.* **2018**, *7*. [CrossRef] [PubMed]
54. Hilgers, R.H.P.; Oparil, S.; Wouters, W.; Coelingh Bennink, H.J.T. Vasorelaxing effects of estetrol in rat arteries. *J. Endocrinol.* **2012**, *215*, 97–106. [CrossRef]
55. Montt-Guevara, M.M.; Giretti, M.S.; Russo, E.; Giannini, A.; Mannella, P.; Genazzani, A.D.A.R.; Genazzani, A.D.A.R.; Simoncini, T. Estetrol modulates endothelial nitric oxide synthesis in human endothelial cells. *Front. Endocrinol.* **2015**, *6*, 111. [CrossRef] [PubMed]
56. Coelingh Bennink, H.J.T.; Verhoeven, C.; Zimmerman, Y.; Visser, M.; Foidart, J.M.; Gemzell-Danielsson, K. Pharmacokinetics of the fetal estrogen estetrol in a multiple-rising-dose study in postmenopausal women. *Climacteric* **2017**, *20*, 285–289. [CrossRef]
57. Raps, M.; Helmerhorst, F.; Fleischer, K.; Thomassen, S.; Rosendaal, F.; Rosing, J.; Ballieux, B.; Van Vliet, H. Sex hormone-binding globulin as a marker for the thrombotic risk of hormonal contraceptives. *J. Thromb. Haemost.* **2012**, *10*, 992–997. [CrossRef] [PubMed]
58. Odlind, V.; Milsom, I.; Persson, I.; Victor, A. Can changes in sex hormone binding globulin predict the risk of venous thromboembolism with combined oral contraceptive pills? *Acta Obstet. Gynecol. Scand.* **2002**, *81*, 482–490. [CrossRef]
59. Coelingh Bennink, H.J.T.; Verhoeven, C.; Zimmerman, Y.; Visser, M.; Foidart, J.M.; Gemzell-Danielsson, K. Pharmacodynamic effects of the fetal estrogen estetrol in postmenopausal women: Results from a multiple-rising-dose study. *Menopause* **2017**, *24*, 677–685. [CrossRef]
60. Gallez, A.; Blacher, S.; Maquoi, E.; Konradowski, E.; Joiret, M.; Primac, I.; Gérard, C.; Taziaux, M.; Houtman, R.; Geris, L.; et al. Estetrol Combined to Progestogen for Menopause or Contraception Indication Is Neutral on Breast Cancer. *Cancers* **2021**, *13*, 2486. [CrossRef]

MDPI
St. Alban-Anlage 66
4052 Basel
Switzerland
Tel. +41 61 683 77 34
Fax +41 61 302 89 18
www.mdpi.com

Journal of Clinical Medicine Editorial Office
E-mail: jcm@mdpi.com
www.mdpi.com/journal/jcm

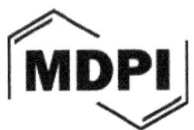

www.ingramcontent.com/pod-product-compliance
Lightning Source LLC
LaVergne TN
LVHW070610100526
838202LV00012B/608